THE DIABETIC COOKBOOK

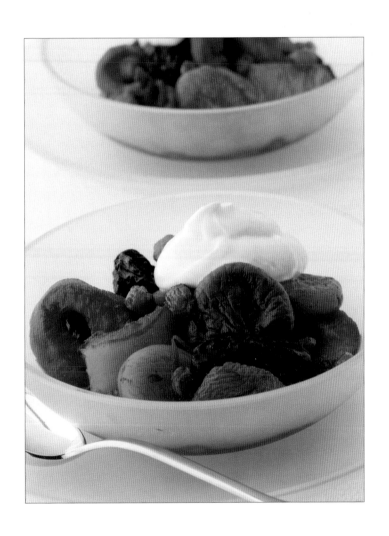

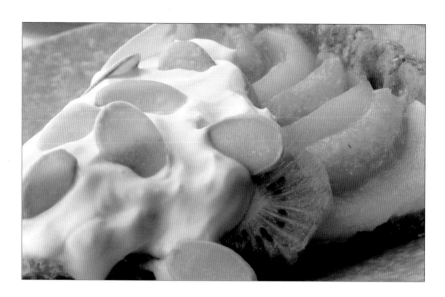

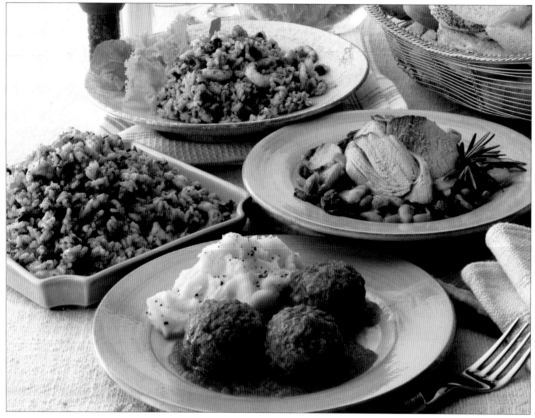

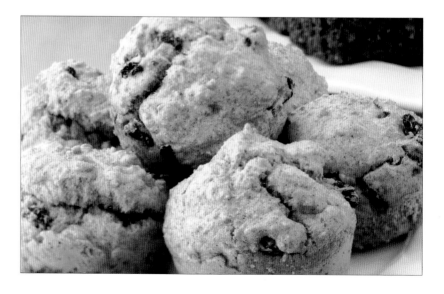

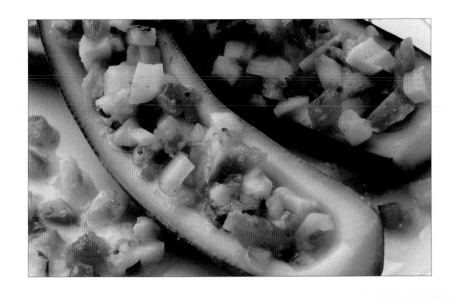

THE DIABETIC COOKBOOK

OVER 50 SUPERB, HIGH-FIBER, LOW-SUGAR RECIPES FOR DIABETICS

MICHELLE BERRIEDALE-JOHNSON

LORENZ BOOKS

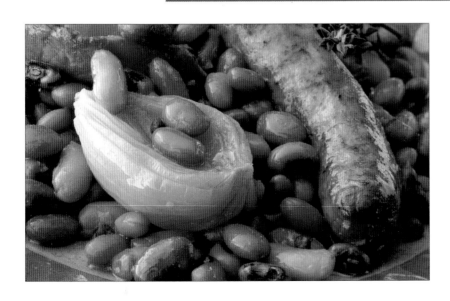

This Paperback edition published by Lorenz Books
27 West 20th Street, New York, NY 10011

LORENZ BOOKS are available for bulk purchase for sales promotion
and for premium use. For details, write or call the sale director,
Lorenz Books, 27 West 20th Street, New York, NY 10011
(800) 354-9657

Lorenz Books is an imprint of Anness Publishing Inc.

ISBN 1 8596 7669 3

Publisher: Joanna Lorenz
Senior Cookery Editor: Linda Fraser
Indexer: Pat Coward
Nutritional Analysis: Helen Daniels
Designer: Ian Sandom
Photography: James Duncan
Food for Photography: Nicola Fowler
Styling: Rosie Hopper

Printed and bound in Singapore

© Anness Publishing Limited 1998
Updated © 1999
3 5 7 9 10 8 6 4 2

NOTES

For all recipes, quantities are given in both metric and imperial measures
and, where appropiate, measures are also given in standard cups and
spoons. Follow one set, but not a mixture, becausethey are not
interchangeable.

Standard spoon and cup measures are level.
1 tsp = 5ml, 1 tbsp = 15ml, 1 cup = 250ml/8fl oz

Australian standard tablespoons are 20ml. Australian readers should
use 3 tsp in place of 1 tbsp for measuring small quantities of gelatine,
cornflour, salt, etc.

Size 3 (medium) eggs are used unless otherwise stated.

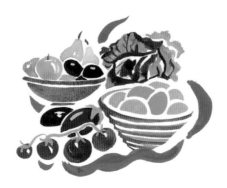

CONTENTS

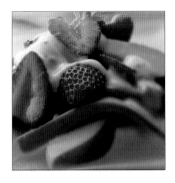
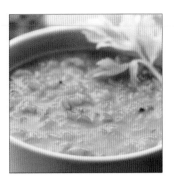

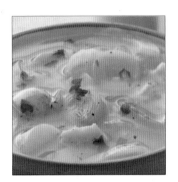
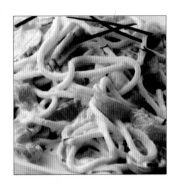
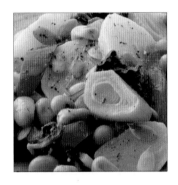
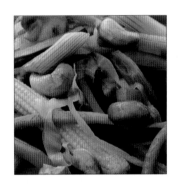
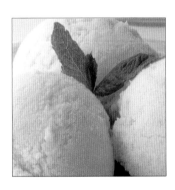
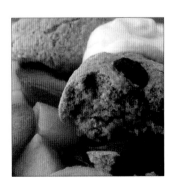

INTRODUCTION

By the time you pick up this book you (or a friend, child or parent) may already have been diagnosed as diabetic, so you should have a pretty good idea of what being diabetic is and what it involves. However, since understanding a situation is often the key to coping with it, it may be worth reviewing the facts about this condition.

Don't be intimidated by the wealth of rather technical information in the next few pages. The principles of dealing with diabetes are really very simple and, once you've got the hang of them, quite easy to cope with.

Most diabetics, especially those recently diagnosed, live very healthy and normal lives—some go on to excel in sports, which many nondiabetics could not dream of. So take heart—and read on.

WHAT IS DIABETES?

The name *diabetes mellitus* comes from two Greek words (*diabetes*–a siphon; *mellitus*–honey, because the urine of a diabetic tastes sweet) and describes a condition in which the sugar (or glucose) circulating in the blood cannot be absorbed properly. This results in abnormally high blood glucose levels, which can cause both short- and long-term problems.

To explain in a bit more detail: Glucose (a form of sugar) is the body's main fuel—it provides us with our energy. We absorb glucose from starchy and sugary carbohydrate foods, such as potatoes, rice and beans, breads, cookies, cakes, sugar and candies. As we chew, enzymes in saliva start breaking down these foods, a process that is continued by the acids in the stomach. As the food progresses on into the gut, digestive juices from the pancreas and gall bladder get to work, and by the time the food reaches the bowel it has been broken down into simple particles (including glucose), which are absorbed through the bowel wall into the bloodstream. The glucose in the bloodstream moves on through the liver, where much of it is stored for future use, and into body cells, where it is either burned up to provide energy or stored for future use.

However, the glucose in the blood cannot enter the cells in the liver or any other part of the body unless a chemical (insulin) effectively "opens the door" into those cells. Insulin is a hormone that is manufactured in the pancreas (the glandular organ that lies behind the stomach but in front of the spine) and stored there until rising glucose levels in the bloodstream set off a chemical reaction that releases the insulin. Once in the bloodstream, the insulin links into the body's cells through what are called insulin receptors (a procedure that is rather like two spaceships docking). This linkage precipitates chemical changes in the cell walls that allow the glucose through into the cell, where it can be converted into energy.

In a nondiabetic this monitoring and replenishment process happens automatically, so that the body's cells are continually fed with sufficient glucose for their energy needs while excess glucose is stored in the cells. In a diabetic the system fails, either because the pancreas does not produce any insulin at all (Insulin Dependent Diabetes or Type I) or because the pancreas's supply of insulin is reduced, the supply of insulin receptors is reduced or neither functions very efficiently (Non-Insulin Dependent Diabetes or Type II).

Despite years of research, no one has discovered why it is that the pancreas should (as in the onset of Type I) suddenly cease to produce insulin, although it would appear that some people can have a genetic predisposition to diabetes. For susceptible individuals, a viral disease can act on the immune system to make it turn on the "beta" cells in the pancreas, which manufacture the insulin, and destroy them. In Type II there seems to be not only a genetic but a radical

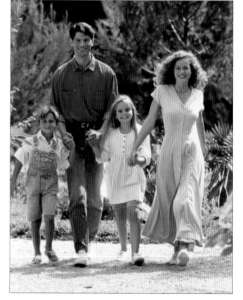

Above: Children and young adults are more likely to be Type I diabetics than Type II diabetics.

predisposition: Type II is four times more common in Asian communities than in the rest of the population in Britain, for example. However, with Type II, which occurs mainly in older and frequently overweight people (Type I usually occurs in thin children and people under 30), there does appear to be a link with obesity. Other possible contributory causes to Type II in later years could be pancreatic damage through surgery or alcohol abuse; glucose intolerance during pregnancy, which may disappear after the baby is born but leaves a predisposition to diabetes during later pregnancies or in later life; long-term use of some steroids, which raise the amount of glucose in the blood; and overactivity of the thyroid.

DIAGNOSIS AND SYMPTOMS

Diagnosis of insulin dependent diabetes is normally fairly straightforward since the symptoms, although varied, are pretty obvious and can even be quite dramatic. Non-insulin dependent diabetes is another matter, since the fall in insulin production may occur over a number of years and the symptoms may be quite slight. Some people with Type II have no symptoms at all.

DIAGNOSIS

If you go to a doctor complaining of any of the symptoms at the far right, he or she will likely check for diabetes.

The first test might be for excess glucose in the urine, although since the glucose levels in the urine tend to fluctuate (and some people have a low threshold and so register as having above the normal level without actually being diabetic), the existence of such an excess is not absolute proof of diabetes. It is more usual to be sent for a blood glucose test. This blood will be taken from a vein, not a finger prick. By the time blood reaches the finger through the small blood vessels or capillaries, it has used up some of the glucose it was originally carrying and does not give an accurate picture. So it is important to measure the glucose in blood taken from a vein (the venous plasma glucose concentration). The normal glucose concentration that you would expect to find, according to World Health Organization (WHO) criteria, is below 7.8mmol/liter.

A diabetic, according to the WHO criteria, is one whose "venous plasma glucose concentration" when he has been fasting, remains at 7.8mmol/liter, but rises to above 11.1mmol/liter on a random blood sample. Between "normal" and "diabetic" they list a third category of those with "impaired glucose tolerance" (7.8mmol/liter fasting and between 7.8 and 11.1mmol/liter on a random test). These people may return to normal, may go on to develop full-blown diabetes or may remain at the same level. They should, however, follow a diabetic regime and keep themselves as healthy as possible.

TREATMENT

Although serious, even Type I has become a treatable condition since the arrival of injectable insulin. Provided you are prepared to adhere to your regime, there is no reason why you should not lead a full life.

The key to the management and treatment of both Type I and Type II is to take over the job normally performed by the insulin in the body and keep your blood sugar levels normal. Allowing them to get too high, or too low, can cause a variety of problems and is to be avoided. This does not mean getting paranoid about blood sugar levels or diet—merely keeping a sensible watch on both.

For Type IIs, a change in diet, possibly in conjunction with medication to lower blood glucose levels, will frequently achieve the desired result. Indeed, changes to the diet may improve the health of an individual to such an extent that the onset of his or her diabetes may be viewed as something of a blessing.

Type Is have benefitted from the development of sophisticated blood-testing techniques. These usually involve taking a drop of blood from the finger or ear lobe and have made it much easier to control blood glucose levels, by changing either the diet or the insulin dose.

Whether you have been diagnosed as being an insulin dependent diabetic or a diabetic who is non-insulin dependent, your doctor will instruct you in the use of your drugs, insulin and glucose testing equipment. He or she will also give you dietary guidance or send you to a dietitian. The principles and practices for a good diabetic diet are described later in this introduction and further amplified in the recipe section.

SYMPTOMS

Thirst (polydipsia) and passing large quantities of urine (polyuria)
If the levels of glucose in the blood are too high, the kidneys no longer filter all the glucose, and some escapes into the urine. The extra glucose thickens the urine; it draws extra water with it to help it to flow through the kidneys, and this causes the bladder to fill. The individual needs to urinate often and in copious amounts. At the same time the body becomes dehydrated, which leads to a terrible thirst.

Constipation
As the body becomes more dehydrated, constipation becomes almost inevitable.

Tiredness and weight loss
Since our bodies acquire their energy from glucose, anyone whose body cannot access the glucose circulating in the blood will be short of energy and therefore tired. In an effort to replace this energy, the body will break down other cells/body tissues, thus causing a weight loss that can be dramatic.

Blurred vision
Excess sugar in the blood makes it thick and syrupy. In some diabetics, this can upset the focusing of the eyes—their vision becomes blurred.

Infections
When the blood becomes thick and syrupy due to the presence of excess glucose, this may also affect the functioning of the immune system. The undiagnosed diabetic may be prone to all kinds of infections, including skin eruptions, urinary tract infections such as thrush or cystitis, and chest infections.

Pins and needles
Changes in the blood glucose levels may also affect nerve functions, resulting in tingling or "pins and needles" in the hands or feet.

ALTERNATIVE THERAPIES

Once the pancreas has given up on insulin production, it can very rarely be "kicked back into action." However, certain alternative or complementary therapies can stimulate pancreatic function, improve the body's insulin response and moderate glucose levels, so they are worth considering both in cases of non-insulin dependent diabetes and in the immediate aftermath of the onset of insulin dependent diabetes, when there may still be some residual function in the pancreas.

Equally important is the diabetic's need to keep as fit and healthy—in both mind and body—as possible. It is recognized that stress does more damage to our health than almost anything else— and that many alternative therapies are very helpful in dealing with stress. Yoga, meditation, reflexology, aromatherapy and massage are the best-known stress relievers, but many people find spiritual healers, color therapists or practicing T'ai Chi just as helpful.

CHINESE MEDICINE

The Chinese have recognized diabetes as a disease for many thousands of years. However, Chinese medicine approaches the body, bodily functions and bodily malfunctions from an entirely different angle than Western medicine. To a Chinese doctor, diabetes is a sign of disharmony in the body, whose symptoms appear in the upper body (raging thirst, dry mouth, drinking huge quantities), middle body (large appetite and excessive eating accompanied by weight loss and constipation) and lower body (copious urination, progressive weight loss, etc.).

Chinese medical treatment would therefore concentrate on restoring the harmony within the individual with the aim of improving the symptoms and addressing the disease.

Even if this approach does not directly affect insulin production or control, improving the body's natural harmony should improve the diabetic's general health and therefore his or her ability to cope well with diabetes. However, insulin dependent diabetics must not change their insulin regime if they attend a Chinese physician, except on the express instruction of their diabetes specialist.

RELAXATION AND MASSAGE THERAPIES

It is recognized that stress plays a significant role in the development of diabetes. Any therapy that reduces stress and helps you to relax is therefore likely to have a beneficial effect on control of your diabetes and on your general health.

Yoga and meditation have been found to have a positive impact on blood glucose levels, while moderate exercise helps insulin work more efficiently in the body.

Reflexology helps to tone and relax the body, and although it cannot address the cause of diabetes, it can alleviate some of the side effects.

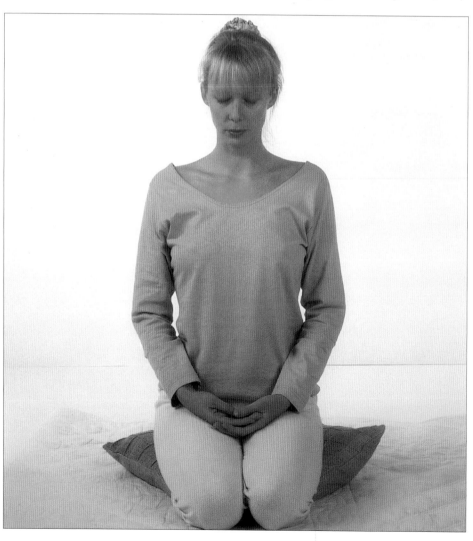

Left: Yoga and meditation are both said to reduce blood glucose levels by helping you relax and reduce stress.

SELF-MASSAGE

Aromatherapy (massage with essential herbal oils) is not only relaxing, but can also improve circulation and therefore help to heal the leg and foot ulcers to which some diabetics are prone.

The therapeutic potential of aromatherapy oils, although recognized in the past, has been largely ignored until recently. However, it is now realized that concentrated oils (made from plants and herbs that filled our ancestors' medicine chests) can be very helpful for many specific complaints.

Essential oils are easily absorbed through the skin into the bloodstream and so are particularly effective for circulatory problems. Some oils, such as hyssop, are good for the circulation as a whole; others, such as grapefruit, lemon, lime, fennel and white birch, are lymphatic stimulants; while spike lavender, rosemary, eucalyptus, peppermint and thyme stimulate sluggish circulation. Massage is a good way to apply essential oils as it is relaxing, and it also ensures that the oils are effectively absorbed.

LEG AND FOOT MASSAGE

Self-massage is relatively easy and can help considerably in reducing stiffness and sluggishness of blood flow in the legs.

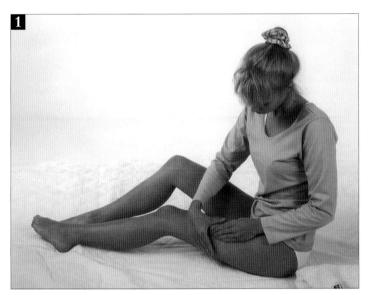

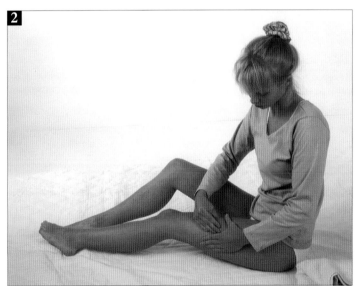

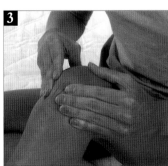

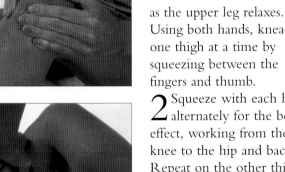

1 Start a leg massage by working on the thighs, so that any fluid in the calves will have somewhere to go as the upper leg relaxes. Using both hands, knead one thigh at a time by squeezing between the fingers and thumb.

2 Squeeze with each hand alternately for the best effect, working from the knee to the hip and back. Repeat on the other thigh.

3 Around the knees, do a similar kneading action but just using the fingers for a lighter effect and working in smaller circles.

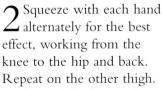

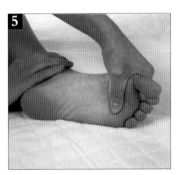

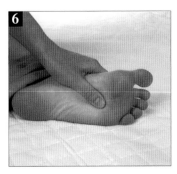

4 Bend your leg, and if possible raise the foot onto a chair or handy ledge. With your thumbs, work on the back of each calf with a circular, kneading action. Repeat this action a few times on each leg, each time working from the ankle up to the knee.

5 Squeeze the foot with your hands, loosening up the muscles and gently stretching the arch.

6 To complete the massage, use firm pressure with your thumb to stretch the foot. Repeat on the other foot.

FOOD AND HERBAL MEDICINES

Certain foods and herbs, although they cannot reinstate pancreatic function, can help the pancreas to function more efficiently. They may also improve the absorption of insulin and lead to better control of glucose levels in the blood by the body and to improved circulation. This may, in part, be due to the nutrients found in these foods and herbs (see Nutritional Medicine, below), but there is increasing scientific evidence that certain foods and herbs have special health-giving properties that cannot be entirely attributed to their vitamin or mineral content.

FOODS WITH HEALTH-GIVING PROPERTIES

• Whole oats, onions, globe artichokes and legumes all have the ability to reduce blood sugar.
• Wheat germ, underripe bananas, turkey, fish, walnuts, red peppers and cruciferous vegetables, such as broccoli and cauliflower (all good sources of Vitamin B_6), help to control blood sugar levels.
• Shellfish, lean meat, whole-grain cereals, legumes, pumpkin seeds and nuts are all high in chromium and zinc (diabetics are commonly deficient in both minerals).
• Blueberries have been found to help in the control of diabetic retinopathy.
• Wheat germ, sunflower seeds, canola oil, almonds and sweet potatoes (all containing high levels of Vitamin E) have been shown to help improve diabetic circulation and neuropathy.
• Fresh nettle juice has been used since Roman times to stimulate the circulation, while common dandelion greens have an equally lengthy pedigree for the stimulation of the liver (where glucose is stored).

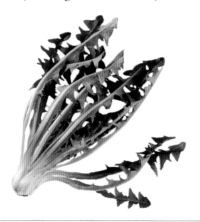

Above: Dandelion greens have been used for centuries as a stimulant for the liver.

NUTRITIONAL MEDICINE

Effects of nutrient deficiencies
Although it has long been recognized that we need a wide range of vitamins and minerals for our bodies to function efficiently, there is a growing belief that many of today's degenerative illnesses, such as diabetes, could be caused by serious deficiencies in micro-nutrients, such as vitamins, minerals and amino acids. These deficiencies, it is argued, have resulted from our eating over-processed foods, living in a highly polluted environment and subjecting ourselves to hitherto unknown levels of stress. Research is going on all the time and continues to reveal links between certain degenerative conditions and particular nutrient deficiencies.

Chromium is an essential trace element. Although it is present only in minute quantities in the body, it appears to be necessary for blood sugar control and the proper action of insulin. Unfortunately, chromium is removed from refined carbohy-drates during processing. Chromium is difficult to take as a supplement but is absorbed from brewer's yeast, black pepper, wheat germ, whole-wheat bread and cheese.

Vitamins B_6 and B_{12} can both help blood sugar control. Vitamin B_{12} levels can be reduced by certain diabetic drugs, so it is useful to include sources of this vitamin (lean meat and dairy products) in the diet.

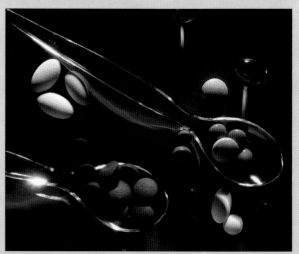

Above: Nutritional supplements can help to ensure that you are getting the right amounts of some vitamins, minerals and essential fatty acids.

Vitamin C is known to strengthen fragile blood capillaries, especially in the eye, and to reduce elevated cholesterol levels—both conditions that affect diabetics.

Zinc, magnesium and potassium are all very important for diabetics, but levels can be seriously depleted through excess urination. Zinc is important for combating infections such as eczema, acne and thrush, many of which afflict diabetics. Magnesium is also important for the proper functioning of the kidneys.

Essential fatty acids There is increasing evidence that a diabetic's absorption of essential fatty acids may be impeded by raised blood sugar or insulin deficiency, so taking a supplement, such as evening primrose oil, may help prevent diabetic complications.

KEEPING BLOOD GLUCOSE LEVELS NORMAL

The ideal state for a diabetic is for blood sugar levels to remain normal. Careful monitoring of these, a good diet and medication where necessary are basic strategies. However, many other aspects of the diabetic's life may impinge on his or her blood sugar levels.

BLOOD GLUCOSE LEVELS

Changing exercise levels, for example, can affect both the efficiency of insulin uptake and the rate at which the sugar in the blood is used up. Stress of any kind may cause an adrenaline release that will increase the level of sugar in the blood. Infections, injuries or operations are felt by the body as stress. The body reacts by releasing adrenaline or other hormones into the bloodstream, and these again push up the sugar levels.

Pregnancy causes changes in blood sugar levels, as do monthly periods and menopause. Medical drugs, especially steroids and some diuretics and anti-depressants, can also affect blood sugar levels. If any of these factors apply, it is essential to monitor your blood sugar levels even more carefully than usual, adapting your diet or adjusting your insulin dose or the levels of the drug you take to lower blood glucose, in consultation with your doctor, if necessary.

Serious fluctuations in glucose levels cause hypoglycemia (too little sugar) and hyperglycemia (too much sugar) and have very specific symptoms, which need to be treated immediately. If dramatic rises (and, more especially, falls) in blood sugar are treated immediately, there are unlikely to be long-term effects. However, persistent slightly raised blood sugar levels of about 8–19mmol/liter do have a number of serious consequences in terms of health.

CORONARY HEART DISEASE

Elevated triglycerides (fats in the blood) are a common feature of poorly controlled diabetes and add greatly to the risk of coronary heart disease (when the arteries supplying blood to the heart "clog up," thus depriving the heart muscle of the blood it needs to function properly), so diabetics need to be particularly careful about eating a low-fat diet and making sure that they are not overweight.

STROKE

High blood pressure is another area that diabetics need to watch. Keeping their weight normal, stopping smoking and eating a low-fat, low-salt diet will usually help a great deal to minimize the risk of strokes.

Below: Pregnancy will affect blood glucose levels, which need to be monitored.

NEUROPATHY

Diabetic neuropathy is very common in long-term and poorly controlled diabetics. Although there are many variations, neuropathy happens when the nerve ends become damaged (as a result of excess glucose flowing through the capillaries or small veins). Neuropathy normally affects the hands and feet (tingling or pins and needles in the hands and feet is one of the symptoms of diabetes) and can, over a period, result in loss of all feeling in the extremities.

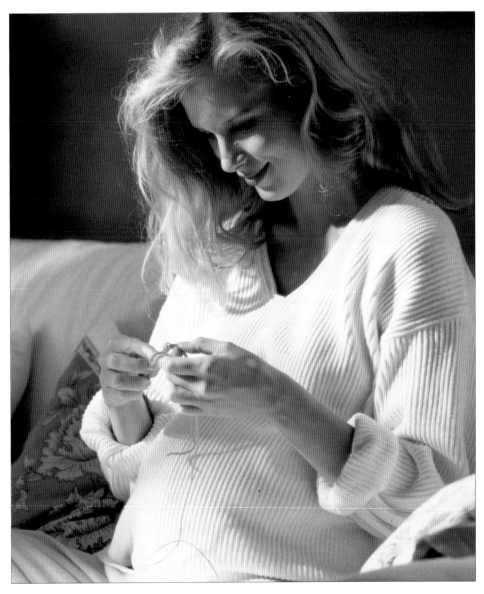

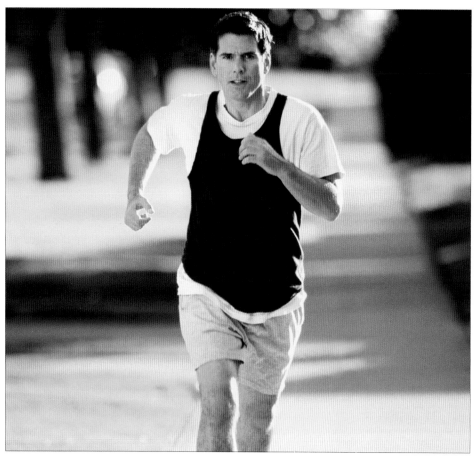

Left: Exercise, such as jogging, increases the rate at which sugar in the blood is used up – to prevent a dangerous dip in your blood glucose level, eat a small carbohydrate snack before, or immediately after, any exercise.

Neuropathy presents two problems. One is that the circulation to the more remote areas of the body gets worse and this can lead to infected wounds, bad healing and, in the worst cases, gangrene. Feet and legs are especially prone to damage and need to be looked after and monitored with great care. The other problem is that the feet lose all sensation. This not only affects balance and the ability to walk properly but also means that the sufferer is at risk of injury, perhaps by being scalded by getting into too hot a bath, because his or her feet have become so insensitive to temperature.

Diabetics can also suffer some damage to their "autonomic nerves." These are the nerves that carry the instructions to the various organs, such as heart, kidneys, bladder and bowels, and tell them what to do. Damage to these autonomic nerves can result in poor bowel or bladder control, failure of the stomach to empty properly and similar problems. Typically all these functions will return to normal when the blood glucose levels have also returned to normal.

KIDNEY AND EYE DAMAGE

The kidneys and the eyes are two areas of the body filled with capillaries or tiny blood vessels that are especially prone to diabetic damage. Excess blood sugar can "clog up" both areas, but whereas kidney damage may be reversed or at least controlled by diet and good blood glucose control, damage to the eyes may be irreversible. Maintaining good control of blood glucose levels will minimize the damage. It is particularly important that diabetics have very regular eye exams and that these include an examination of the retina.

SKIN PROBLEMS

Because raised blood sugar makes one more prone to infection, especially skin infection, badly controlled diabetes will often result in boils, pimples, and rashes. Most of these will respond well to good diet and improved control.

This disturbing list of symptoms may sound like a life sentence, but diabetics should remember that most of them only occur when they do not look after themselves. These days, a diabetic diet is almost identical to the healthy diet recommended for all of us – so the diabetic need not be singled out as an oddity. Because of the huge improvement in both monitoring and injection techniques, even insulin dependent diabetics can check their blood sugar levels and administer their insulin both quickly and discreetly. However, this does not mean that you should keep your diabetes a secret. For a start, there is no reason to, as you can live a perfectly full life with diabetes. Second, friends, colleagues and even strangers need to know that you are diabetic in case you suffer a hyper- or hypoglycemic attack. This is easily dealt with, but very frightening if you or others do not know what is going on. Consider wearing a diabetic identification bracelet or tag.

All diabetes does require is that you take it seriously and be organized about dealing with it. You must be rigorous about checking your glucose levels, you must always make sure that you have your insulin or drugs available and you must always make sure that you have extra glucose or carbohydrate food should you need it. Finally, you must be aware that your body is more sensitive to change than that of someone without diabetes, so you must pay attention to what it tells you in terms of "feeling different" or unwell. Your body is the best possible monitor of its own condition, so it is important to listen to it!

HYPER- AND HYPOGLYCEMIA

Hyper- and hypoglycemia occur when blood sugar levels rise too high (hyper) or fall too low (hypo).

HYPERGLYCEMIA

The symptoms of hyperglycemia are usually less dramatic than those of hypoglycemia, but because tissue damage may result if the blood sugar levels remain too high (usually over 11–12mmol/liter), it is important to get the levels down quickly.

Elevated levels of blood sugar can be the result of uncontrolled long-term diabetes, but there can also be more immediate causes. Forgetting to take your insulin or blood glucose drugs will cause your blood sugar levels to rise, as will eating much more than you usually do—or eating a fattier or more sugary meal than normal.

Reducing the amount of exercise you usually take could affect glucose levels. An infection, illness, operation or accident could all cause blood sugar levels to rise, as can pregnancy and menstruation. Careful monitoring will reveal the raised levels quickly—anything over 11mmol/liter is undesirable—and changes in insulin, drugs or diet should get you back to normal.

HYPOGLYCEMIA

Hypoglycemia can occur in non-diabetics whose blood sugar levels fall too low; the official definition is below 2.5mmol/liter. However, this reaction is most often seen in diabetics who have taken more insulin than they need or have eaten too little—or exercised too much—relative to their last dose of insulin or glucose-lowering drugs.

Although the symptoms of hypoglycemia can be dramatic, the results are seldom serious, and it is extremely easy to treat. All you need is a rapid intake of sugar in the form of glucose tablets (Dextrose, Dextro), sugar cubes, honey, candy, fruit juice or cookies. Even when the symptoms are quite extreme, the diabetic will be back to normal in a matter of minutes.

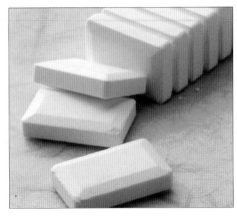

Above: Glucose tablets are a simple and speedy remedy for mild hypoglycemia.

However, he or she then needs to back up the instant injection of glucose with more solid food, as the excess insulin will quickly absorb the initial blast of glucose and will need something further to work on.

The problem with hypoglycemia is that the brain is utterly dependent on an adequate supply of glucose to function properly. The first sign that a diabetic is suffering from a "hypo" may be a failure in his or her logical reasoning powers. This can manifest itself as a refusal to accept that he may be suffering from a hypo—which is why it is particularly important for friends and colleagues to know that he is diabetic (and for the diabetic to carry a card or consider wearing an identifying bracelet or badge), so that if his hypo symptoms take the form of denial, someone else can get a glucose tablet into his mouth.

Hypo symptoms vary enormously, but they often include lack of concentration, difficulty in making even simple decisions or a feeling of being confused. A common feeling is that you must finish whatever you are doing, even though you are feeling odd. This is particularly dangerous if you are driving a car, so diabetics must make every effort to recognize and combat this compulsion.

Hypos can often cause behavioral changes and quite violent mood swings. Coordination may also be impaired. They may stagger as if drunk and have difficulty in performing the simplest task—like unwrapping a glucose tablet!

If unrecognized and untreated, a hypo will eventually cause a diabetic to lose consciousness, but even then an injection of glucagon (the antidote to insulin) will bring the diabetic around to the point where he or she can be fed a proper dose of glucose.

Since symptoms are so varied, it is important that diabetics be aware of changes in their physical or mental states, that they monitor their blood sugar levels regularly, compensate for any changes in their daily routine and always carry glucose tablets (or the equivalent) with them. Long-term diabetics should be aware that over time symptoms of hypo decrease, so that their blood sugar may fall without them having any symptoms at all.

A FEW WORDS OF WARNING

• Ignore rising blood sugar levels at your peril. Your body's reaction will not be as rapid as with low levels, but if ignored rising blood sugar levels can put you into a coma.

• Never give up your insulin or drug regime—even if you are vomiting. The greater the stress on the body, the greater its need for insulin to combat rising blood sugar levels. Vomiting is serious for a diabetic, so maintain your drug regime and consult a doctor.

• Because the body is infinitely adaptable, some people will feel quite ill when their blood sugar is only slightly raised, while others will still feel relatively okay with seriously high levels. Moreover, long-term undiagnosed diabetics may have gotten used to having high levels of sugar in their blood, so they will not even notice feeling ill.

• It is particularly important to monitor your blood sugar levels on a regular basis, even if you feel fine.

HEALTHY EATING

Diet is the backbone of both insulin dependent and non-insulin dependent diabetic management, and the first line of attack in stabilizing blood sugar control. Today, the diabetic diet varies little from the diet that everyone should be eating: to eat at least five portions of fruit and vegetables each day, to take in less than 30 percent of calories from fat (with most of it coming from mono- and polyunsaturated fats), to reduce the intake of salt (sodium) and sweet foods and to eat plenty of fiber.

THE "OLD" APPROACH

Because sugar is derived from carbohydrates, when the mechanism of carbohydrate absorption was less well understood than it is today, it was thought that diabetics should avoid all carbohydrates. This meant that they had to live on a high-protein, high-fat diet and suffer the side effects, such as high blood pressure, now associated with such a diet. Moreover, a high-fat diet caused them to gain weight.

Below: Protein is needed for growth and cell repair—whole-grain rice, beans, lentils, tofu and walnuts are all good sources.

TODAY'S APPROACH

Research over the last 25 years has turned this thinking on its head, and although present-day diabetics still have to monitor their diet and their carbohydrate intake fairly carefully, they are now encouraged to eat plenty of the right kind of carbohydrate foods, while even a small amount of sugar as such is no longer entirely out of the question.

The food that we eat is made up of proteins, fats, carbohydrates, fiber, micronutrients (vitamins and minerals) and water. The last four (fiber, vitamins, minerals and water) are all essential for the proper functioning of the body, but they do not provide us with energy as such (measured in calories). This we need to get from proteins, fats and carbohydrates.

PROTEINS

Proteins (found in legumes, soy products, nuts, cereals, meat, fish and dairy products) are essential for growth in children and for cell repair in adults. We need to get up to 20 percent of our daily energy intake in the form of proteins.

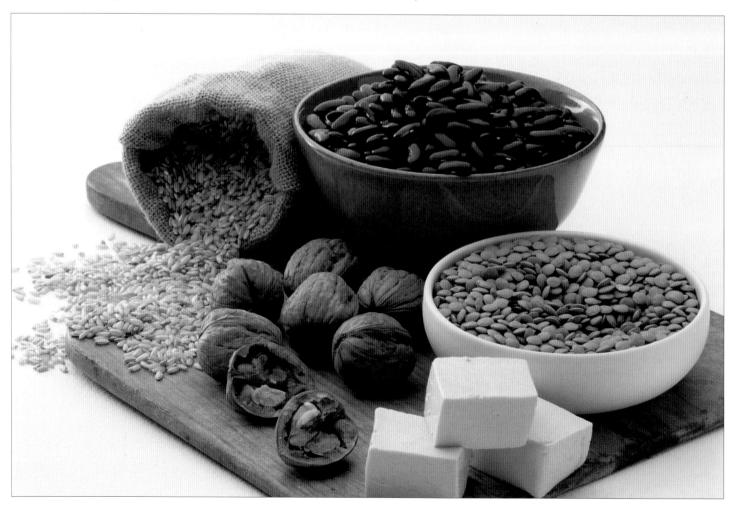

FATS

Fats (found primarily in meat and dairy products, but also in vegetable and fish oils and nuts) are essential to the proper functioning of the body. However, we need the right kind of fat and the right amount. The average Western diet contains far too much of the "wrong" kind of fat—saturated—which leads to obesity, heart problems and strokes. The recommended maximum number of daily calories that should come from fat is between 30 and 35 percent. Unfortunately many Westerners obtain well over 40 percent of their calories from fat.

Fats are broken down into saturated fats (mainly from the fat in meat, but also from dairy products, such as cream, full-fat milk, butter and cheese) and the healthier choices: polyunsaturated fats and mono-unsaturated fats (from vegetable oils, such as olive oil and sunflower oil, and fish oils).

The subject of fats is a very complex one, but for the purposes of the diabetic diet the main thing to remember is that saturated fats are to

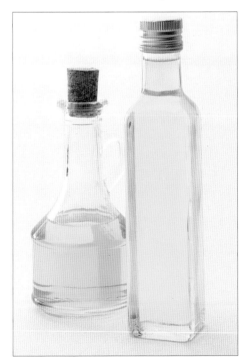

Above: Sunflower oil (left) contains mostly polyunsaturated fats, while olive oil is made up of mainly monounsaturated fats.

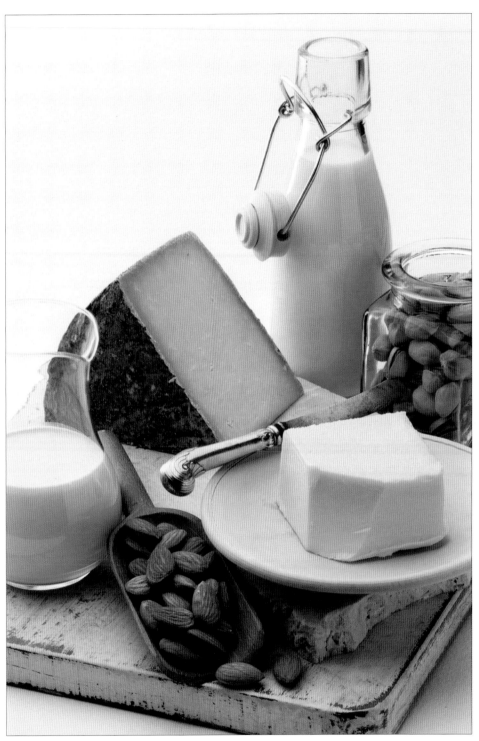

be avoided. These are more likely to cause excess cholesterol to be deposited in the arteries, and because they are higher in calories, obesity is a likely outcome. Diabetics may have high fat concentrations in their blood anyway (making them more vulnerable to arteriosclerosis), so they should avoid making these levels even higher.

Above: Many different foods, such as (clockwise from top right) milk, pistachio nuts, butter, almonds, cream and cheese, contain fats. Dairy products, such as cheese, butter and milk, are sources of saturated fats, which should be avoided by diabetics, while foods such as nuts are good sources of polyunsaturated fats, which, like mono-unsaturated fats, are much more beneficial.

CARBOHYDRATES

Carbohydrates (known in "diet-speak" as CHOs) also come in different guises—simple and complex.

Simple (refined or sugary) carbohydrates consist of various forms of what we know broadly as sugar, or sucrose. In fact, sucrose is made up of glucose and fructose (fruit sugar). Both are essential for providing us with energy, but glucose is particularly important, as the brain depends upon it to function efficiently.

Complex carbohydrates (unrefined carbohydrates) are found in starchy foods such as legumes (beans), oats, rice, potatoes and bread. Complex carbohydrates are made up of simple carbohydrates, glucose (see above) and fiber. The substance known as fiber may be soluble or insoluble. Soluble fiber is found in legumes; it breaks down into a sort of gluey solution, which contains the carbohydrate. Insoluble fiber, such as that found in bran and such vegetables as celery and cabbage, has no nutritional value but is used by the body to move food through the digestive system and to push out what is not wanted as waste.

Once they enter the digestive system, complex carbohydrates are broken down by the digestive juices into their component parts—sucrose and fiber. For a diabetic, the virtue of a carbohydrate made up of sucrose and soluble fiber (legumes) is that the gluey solution into which the soluble fiber turns prevents the system from absorbing the glucose too fast, thus giving the diabetic's impaired glucose-handling system more time to absorb it. The disadvantage of simple carbohydrates (sugar or sucrose) is that they are absorbed almost immediately into the bloodstream, causing sudden glucose "peaks."

Although studies suggest that if it is eaten along with lots of starchy, high-fiber carbohydrate, a small amount of pure sugar can be successfully absorbed by some diabetics without creating glucose peaks, medical advice would still be to avoid sugar whenever possible. "Sugar" in this context would include sugar itself (in tea or coffee, etc.), confections and candies, jams and jellies, cake and cookies sweetened with sugar or fructose, and sweetened carbonated drinks.

"DIABETIC" FOODS

Medical advice is also to avoid expensive proprietary diabetic foods. Although their actual sucrose content may be lower than that of the foods they are meant to replace, they may use fructose or sorbitol as sweeteners (there is little medical evidence that fructose is any better for diabetics than glucose, and sorbitol can cause bowel problems if eaten in large quantities). Finally, these foods may make up for their low sugar content by having a high fat content!

Below: Unrefined, or complex carbohydrates, which are found in such foods as (clockwise from top right) whole-wheat bread, potatoes, oats, beans, and lentils, are absorbed more slowly into the bloodstream.

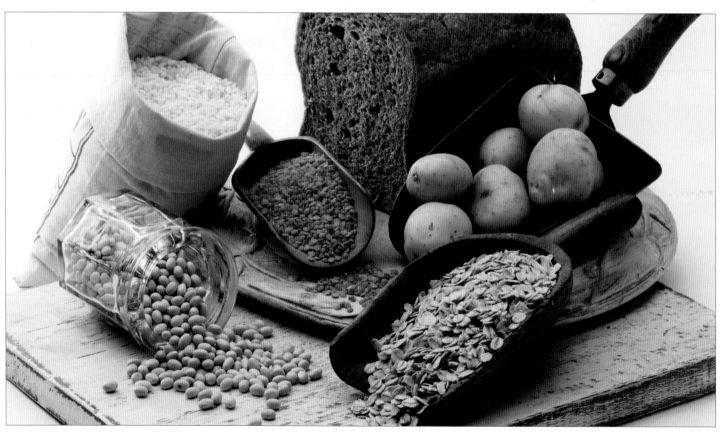

THE DIABETIC'S DAY-TO-DAY DIET

The first thing that the diabetic must remember is that, because the body's ability to absorb sugar is impaired, the system must never be "overloaded." In practice, this means that he or she should have three regularly spaced, moderately sized meals, usually breakfast, lunch and dinner, with two or three regular snacks in between, such as a midmorning and midafternoon snack and a snack at bedtime. For an insulin dependent diabetic the meals must be timed to come 15–30 minutes after the insulin injection so that the insulin has had time to be absorbed into the bloodstream and is ready to cope with the food.

If you are a newly diagnosed diabetic and have led a rather disorganized life, you may find forcing yourself to stick to specific times for meals difficult, but it will prove to be well worth it. And you can console yourself with the thought that if the rest of us ate on a more regular basis we would all feel a lot better, too!

BALANCE

A diabetic should try to make sure that each meal or snack is balanced to include proteins, fats and carbohydrates. This is not difficult to achieve, as many snacks naturally contain all three components in varying amounts. A ham sandwich, for example, includes protein (ham), fat (butter, spread) and carbohydrate (bread).

It is important that the diabetic not miss out on any one element, especially the carbohydrate. Diabetics used to be given a list of what were known as "carbohydrate exchanges," which allocated a carbohydrate value to each food. They then had to figure out how much carbohydrate was in each meal they ate, allocate their meal allowance of carbohydrate and devise a "swap" system if they wanted to change any element of this diet. Today, although diabetic practitioners still allot a total carbohydrate allowance to be spread over the day (based on the diabetic's personal lifestyle, eating patterns, medication, etc.), this does not need to be as rigid as the old exchange system.

AVOIDING EXCESSIVE CALORIE INTAKE

Whereas insulin dependent diabetics are often very thin, non-insulin diabetics, especially long-term ones, tend toward obesity—partly of course because the traditional diabetic diet was high in fat and protein. However, it is very important for diabetics to keep their weight down so as to minimize circulatory and other diseases.

As anyone knows who has tried to diet, the only long-term answer is to reduce the total amount of food that you eat and to change the nature of that food.

Reducing the amount of sugar in your diet will set you well on the way; reducing the amount of fat, especially saturated fat, in your diet will help even more. And reduction does not necessarily mean total deprivation!

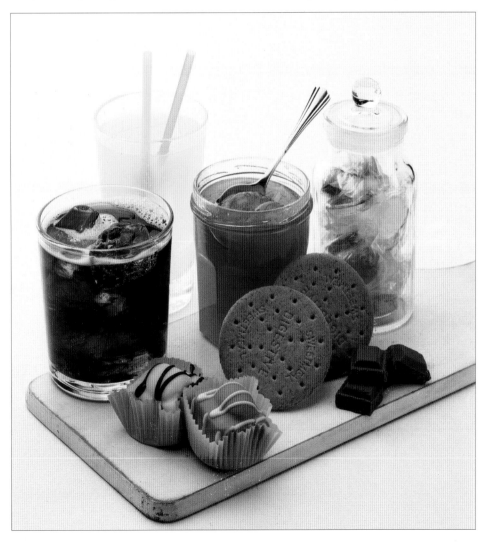

Right: Carbonated, sweetened drinks, full-sugar jam, cookies, candies, chocolate and cakes aren't completely banned, but consumption of these high-calorie foods should be kept to a minimum.

REDUCING SUGAR

Most diabetic practitioners would prefer their patients to stop sweetening their tea and coffee. However, if the thought is too terrible to contemplate, intense sweeteners, such as aspartame (NutraSweet) or saccharin (Sweet 'n' Low) are better than sugar, but their consumption should be kept to a minimum.

Sugar in drinks other than coffee and tea—carbonated drinks, colas, etc.—should be avoided. Not only do these drinks give an instant glucose hit (bad for diabetic control), but they are also very caloric (the average cola contains the equivalent of seven teaspoons of sugar). Carbonated water or fresh fruit juice diluted with water are preferable—or, if desperate, the diabetic should stick with low-calorie, artificially sweetened sodas.

Sugar in baking can almost always be replaced with dried or fresh fruits, as is amply illustrated in the recipes that follow. Although fruit contains fructose, this is buried in fibrous flesh, so it is absorbed much more slowly into the system. Fruit also gives a far better flavor to cakes and desserts than granulated sugar, which may be sweet but has no flavor of its own.

Diabetics, indeed all dieters, should also scrutinize labels for added sugar.

Below: Avoid sweetened drinks and opt instead for carbonated water or fresh fruit juice diluted with water.

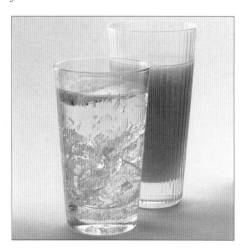

Sometimes this is easy to avoid—buy fruits canned in fruit juice instead of syrup, for example—but it is not always that clear. Remember that on an ingredients list products such as sucrose, fructose, glucose, maltose, honey, lactose, malt and invert corn syrup are all sugar under different names.

Candy and chocolate bars are to be avoided except as a snack before or after exercise. Like sweetened soft drinks, these not only deliver an instant glucose "hit," but they are very high in calories. If total deprivation is not to be borne, try buying chocolate, for example, in thin tablets or drops. It is amazing how satisfying even a morsel of chocolate can be if you nibble it rather than wolfing down a whole bar!

If an apple does not fill that sweet gap, try a few raisins or dates.

They are just as sweet as a mint or a bar of chocolate, but the sugar they contain is embedded in fiber.

Below: To avoid sugar, choose fruits canned in fruit juice, and try apples, dates and raisins as an alternative snack.

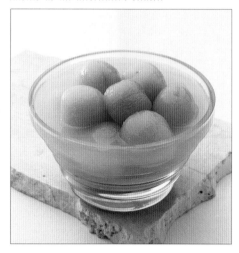

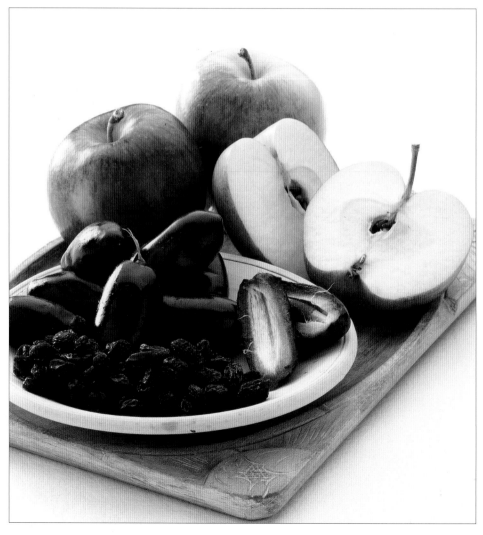

REDUCING FATS

Reducing the amount of calories from fat—especially saturated fat—will help greatly in overall weight control and will also fit in with the specifically diabetic diet. Again, it need not be that difficult to achieve: Some of the new low-fat spreads are really very palatable and work splendidly in pastry and baking. Does a sandwich always need butter or a spread? A ham sandwich with mustard needs neither; a cheese sandwich tastes as good, if not better, with a little low-fat mayonnaise and a lettuce leaf as it does with a thick layer of butter.

Use extra-virgin olive oil or sunflower oil, not butter or vegetable shortening for cooking—and try to limit even that. Meat and vegetables for stews do not need to be fried at the beginning of cooking. If they are cooked long and slowly enough, they will have plenty of flavor. If the occasional plate of French fries is a must, use the oven-ready ones, which have a substantially lower fat content. Ideally the fries should be abandoned in favor of a baked potato—but a baked potato filled with canned tuna and corn, or canned chili or baked beans, not with piles of butter or cheese!

Like French fries, potato chips should really be on the forbidden list. Not only are they caloric and high in fat (even the low-fat ones), but they are very salty—and everyone should be reducing their salt intake! Nuts or (even better) seeds, such as sunflower or pumpkin, maybe lightly salted, are just as good with a drink or as a snack and are very much more nutritious.

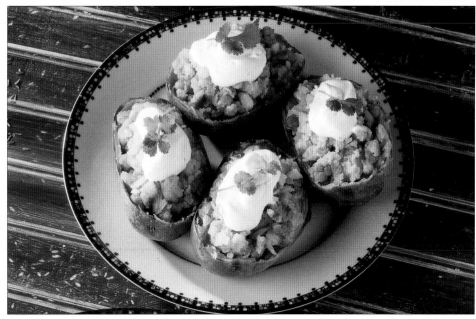

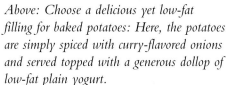

Above: Choose a delicious yet low-fat filling for baked potatoes: Here, the potatoes are simply spiced with curry-flavored onions and served topped with a generous dollop of low-fat plain yogurt.

USING WHOLE-WHEAT BREADS AND FLOURS

Even devoted white bread fans, if they persevere with whole-wheat breads, will find that although whole-wheat breads are not as soft, they have much more flavor. The same applies to using whole-wheat flour in baking. The pastry may not be quite as light, but it will be much more flavorful. There are several other flours that can be used for "lighter but healthier" baking, the most successful of which is gram flour or besan. This is used a lot in Indian cooking. For a diabetic, it has the advantage of being made from a legume, so it is filled with soluble fiber. Gram flour can be substituted for white flour in most instances, and although the pastry will be a little crumbly, it will taste delicious.

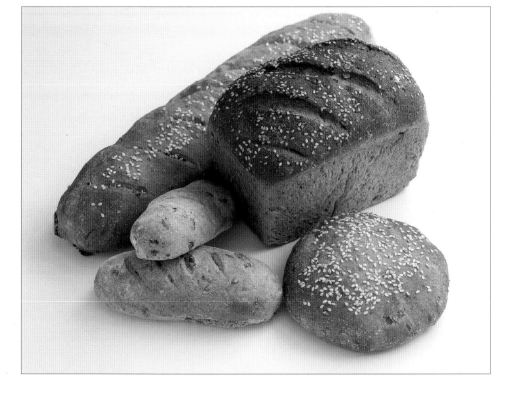

Left: Whole-wheat bread is a healthier option than white bread. However, olive-oil breads, such as ciabatta flavored with olives or sun-dried tomatoes, are better than highly processed sliced white breads.

FILLING YOURSELF UP

The best way to prevent yourself from nibbling—or having the urge to nibble—is by filling yourself up! Try eating large platefuls of colorful salad greens and raw vegetables or lightly cooked vegetables (most of which, being low in fat and carbohydrate, are on the "eat as much as you like" list for diabetics). For a main meal, bulk out vegetables and salads with cooked whole-wheat rice, pasta or cooked beans and pep them up with plenty of chopped fresh herbs and a simple, tasty dressing made from lemon juice and extra-virgin olive oil. It is amazing how satisfying they are. Because the food is full of fiber it will take some time for the body to digest, so that feeling of fullness will not have worn off within half an hour as it so often does after overindulging on Danish pastries.

MONITORING FAT, SODIUM AND FIBER INTAKES

Diabetics who do not need to lose weight still need to monitor their fat, sodium (salt) and fiber intakes. It is very important that diabetics keep the cholesterol levels in their blood under control to limit the risk of coronary heart disease. They should also keep their blood pressure down. A healthy low-fat, low-salt, high-fiber diet will do all of these things—and give a marvelous feeling of well-being.

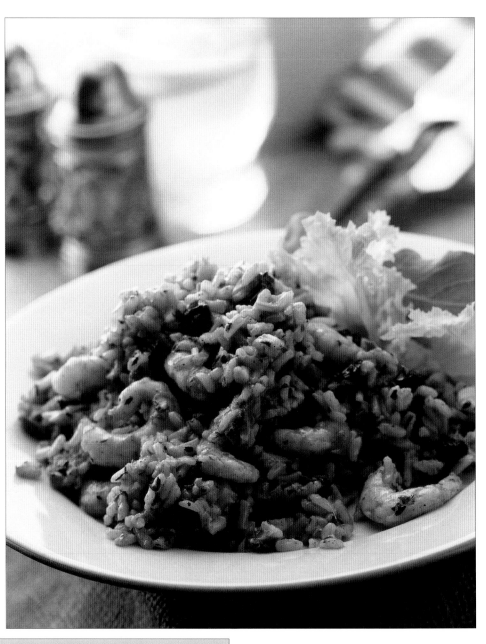

Above: This pilaf of cooked brown rice combined with plenty of lightly cooked vegetables and shrimp is a good example of a satisfying—yet low-fat—meal.

TIPS FOR CUTTING CALORIES

• Using a slightly smaller plate so that a smaller portion still looks generous is an old, but very successful, trick!

• Chewing rather than gulping one's food is another. Some experts recommend up to 20 "chews" per mouthful, but even eight or nine will extend the eating period so that the food seems to go further.

• If the weight still refuses to come off, keep a food diary, in which all food consumed is written down.

• Don't con yourself into thinking that you are sticking to a diet, if you forget about the broken cookie you ate because it fell out of the package, the chunk of cheese you ate while grating a piece for a recipe, the half sausage the children had left on their plates or the lick of the jam spoon as it went into the diswasher.

• Cutting out these few unnecessary calories mentioned above may be all that it takes for the required amount of weight to be lost.

MODERATION

It is very easy, especially for a newly diagnosed diabetic, to get paranoid about his or her diet. This is not only unnecessary but is positively unhelpful: All this does is raise stress levels, and it is well recognized that stress is more debilitating for a diabetic than for anyone else.

FOODS TO EAT AND FOODS TO AVOID

It is very important for diabetics to keep to their overall diet, but the occasional "fall from grace" is not likely to be catastrophic, especially if it can be compensated for at the next meal.

At first it may be hard to remember what is and what is not allowed, but this will soon become second nature. Comparing calorie values is an easy way to monitor general food intake, but it is even more useful to memorize the following categories of foods as early as possible.

FREE FOODS

These can be eaten whenever and in whatever quantity you want.

- all green and leafy vegetables
- cruciferous vegetables (cauliflower, broccoli, turnips, cabbage, etc.)
- salad vegetables (tomatoes, peppers, cucumbers, etc.)
- all members of the onion family
- green peas and green beans
- mushrooms
- fruits, such as raspberries, cranberries and pears
- tea, coffee, water, tomato juice (in moderation), clear soups

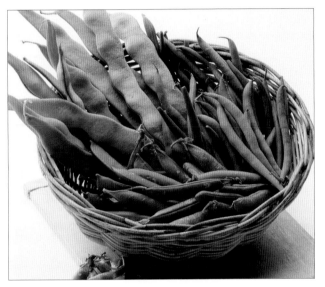

Left: Eat as much as you like—there's no restriction on the quantity of fresh green beans and peas that diabetics can eat.

Below: Fruits, such as (clockwise from top) pears, grapes, nectarines, raspberries and plums, must be counted as part of a diabetic's daily carbohydrate allocation, but make ideal between-meal snacks as well as instant high-fiber desserts.

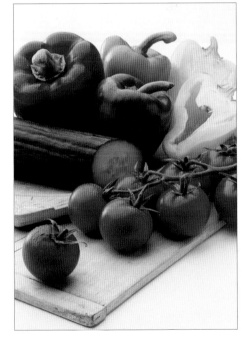

Above: Salad vegetables, such as fresh tomatoes, cucumbers and a variety of colorful peppers, can be eaten in whatever quantity you want—they are very low in sugar, fat and calories, yet are a good source of micronutrients.

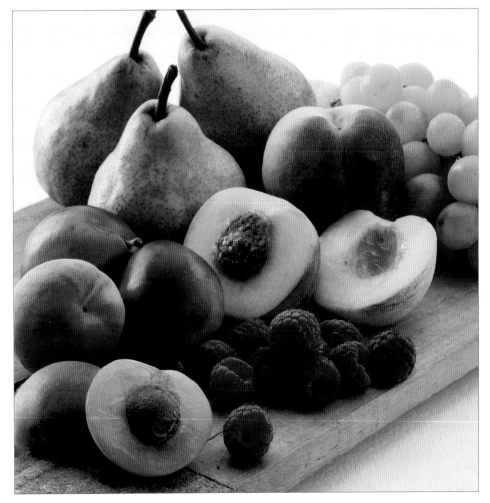

GOOD CARBOHYDRATE/ PROTEIN FOODS

These are good for diabetics to eat, but must be counted as part of an overall carbohydrate and protein allocation.

- all legumes
- brown rice and whole-wheat pasta
- oats, whole-wheat flours, whole-wheat breads and crackers, etc.
- all root vegetables
- all fresh fruits
- all canned fruits as long as canned in unsweetened fruit juice, not syrup
- dried fruits
- high-fiber unsweetened breakfast cereals
- lean poultry, meats or meat products
- fresh and frozen fish
- low-fat cheese, skim milk, low-fat yogurt
- all unsweetened soy products

Right: Soybeans and tofu are good foods for diabetics to eat; however, soy margarine, a healthy alternative to butter, is still a fat and should be used sparingly.

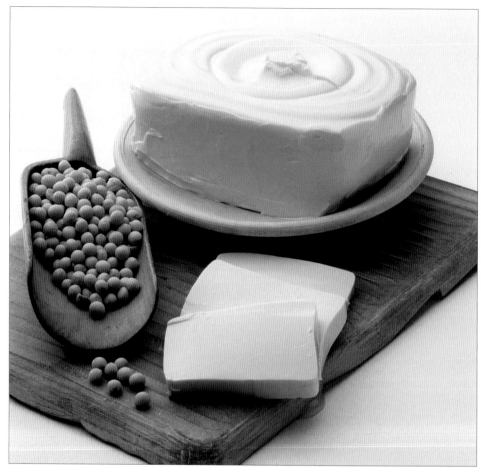

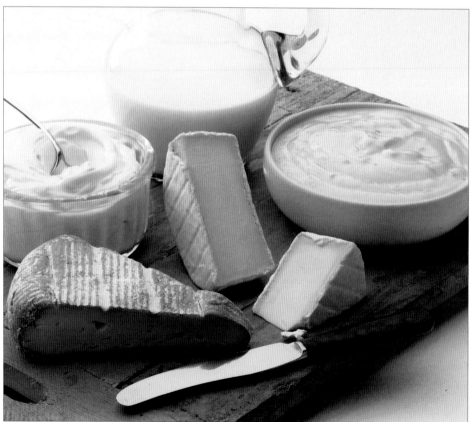

BORDERLINE FOODS

This list reflects less "good" carbohydrate foods and fatty foods—all right to have sometimes in specific quantities, but not ones to overindulge in.

- white flour, white bread, crackers, pastry, white rice and regular pasta
- cornstarch, arrowroot, semolina
- unsweetened breakfast cereals
- any fried potato products, such as French fries and potato chips
- full-fat cheese, cream, full-fat milk, yogurt
- fatty meats, including sausages
- salty meats and fish products
- fruit juices
- reduced-sugar jams, marmalade and other spreads
- alcohol

Left: Borderline foods, such as (clockwise from top) full-fat milk, full-fat sweetened yogurts, full-fat cheeses and cream, can be eaten occasionally, but don't overindulge!

BAD FOODS

These are to be avoided whenever possible and, when eaten, only to be consumed in very small quantities.

- sugar: refined, raw; also honey and corn syrup
- candies, chocolate
- full-sugar chewing gum
- full-sugar jams, marmalades and similar spreads
- cookies, cakes and pastries made with white flour and sugar
- desserts made with refined flours and refined sugar

- fruit canned in syrup
- ice cream and popsicles
- fruit sodas, sweetened drinks, sweetened carbonated drinks
- sweetened breakfast cereals

Below: No longer banned entirely, but sweet treats, such as (clockwise from top left) corn syrup, granulated sugar, honey, confectioners' sugar and raw sugar should only be eaten in small quantities.

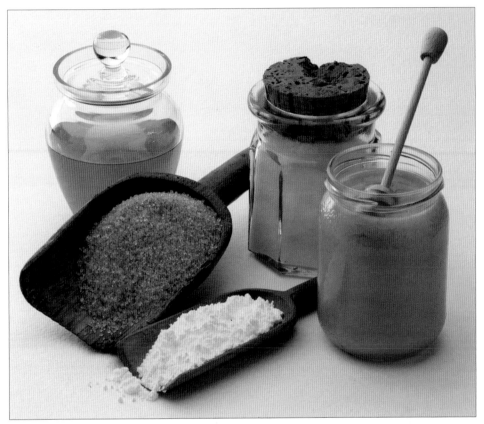

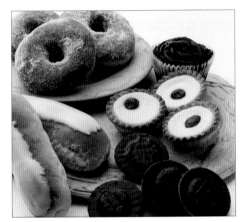

Above: Cookies, cakes and pastries are best avoided by diabetics.

ALCOHOL

Alcohol, such as red wine and beer (*right*), is not entirely off limits for diabetics but must be taken in moderation and calculated into the diet. Beware of low-alcohol drinks. Because less of the sugar has been converted to alcohol, they may contain more sugar. Conversely, low-sugar drinks may contain more alcohol! Remember that alcohol is caloric; if you

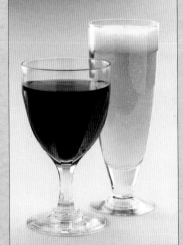

are trying to lose weight, keep your consumption low. It is also important to remember that excess alcohol consumption puts a strain on the liver and the pancreas—both organs that are already under pressure in a diabetic.

ABOUT THE RECIPES

We hope that the recipes in this collection will give diabetics (and non-diabetics) ideas for other dishes that will fulfill the diabetic diet criteria. Any good cookbook should encourage experimentation, so feel free to change—or indeed improve—the recipes that follow.

Our aim has been to introduce ingredients high in soluble fiber, such as legumes, and low in fats and sugars, combined with other more familiar ingredients.

Many of the main-course dishes add lentils or dried beans to meat and vegetables. The only oil used in savory dishes is olive oil or sunflower oil. All baking is done with low-fat spreads and natural fruit sweeteners (apart from the occasional chocolate treat). Those who have never cooked with dried or fresh fruit purées will be amazed at how good the results are—and how little they miss the sugar.

Sodium Levels – Regular bouillon cubes can be very high in salt, so look for "natural" or "organic" bouillon cubes with no added salt. Whenever possible, buy "no added salt or sugar" canned beans and vegetables.

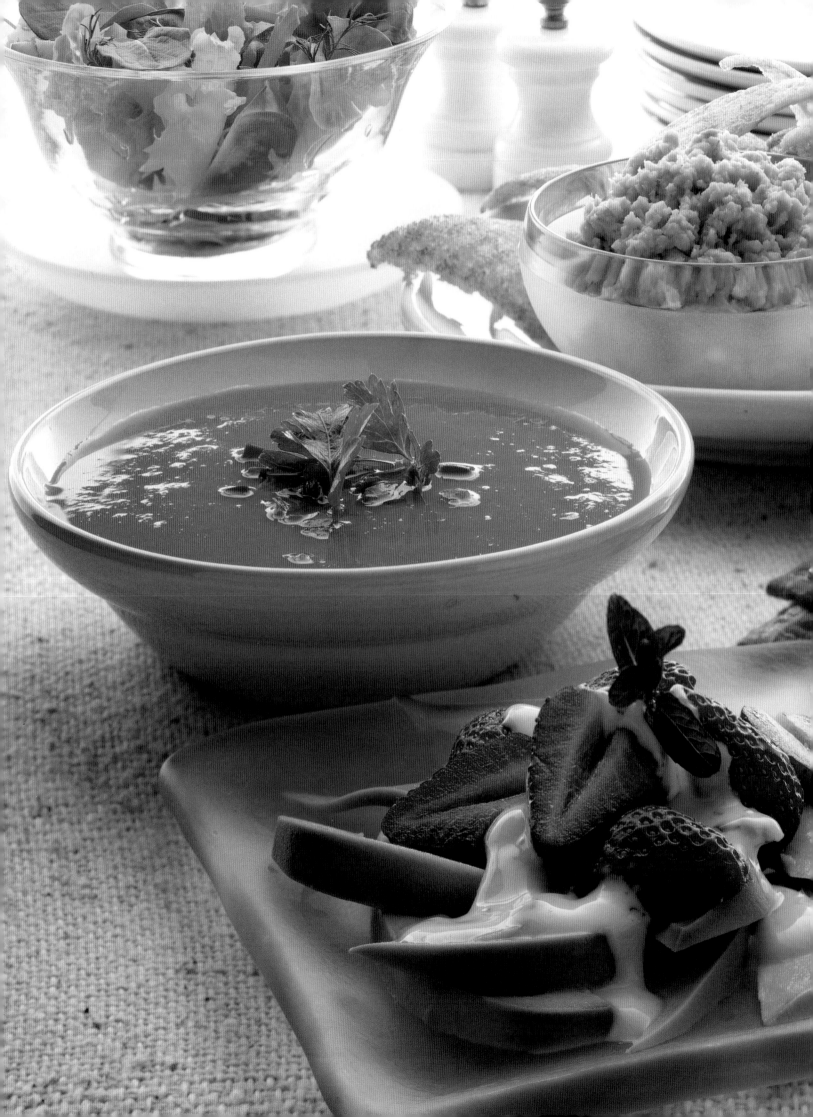

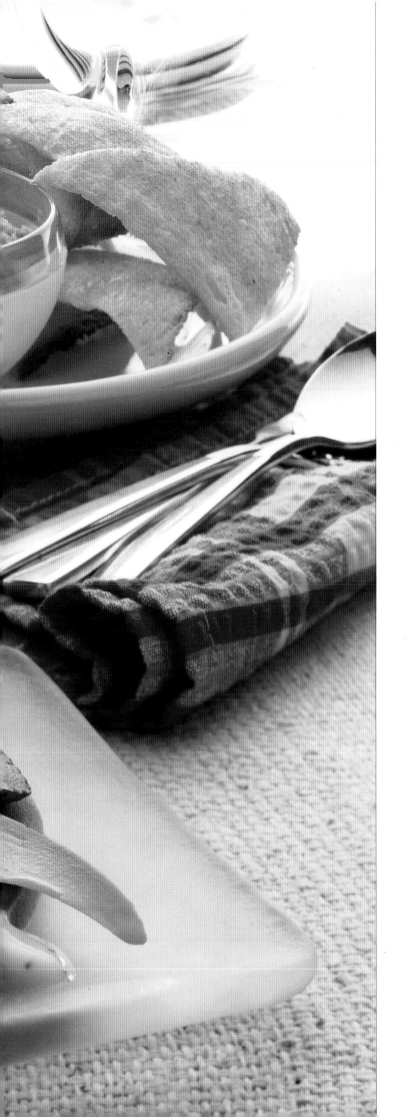

APPETIZERS AND SOUPS

*Vegetable-based appetizers and soups
are ideal for diabetics since they are
often low in fat and sugar and high in
fiber. What is more, it is easy to make
them appealing to the whole family.
This colorful and tasty collection
includes a delectable salad made with
avocados and strawberries, tender
zucchini stuffed with a piquant tomato
and herb salsa, and a range of
stunning soups made with vibrant
vegetables and legumes.*

Chilled Stuffed Zucchini

Full of flavor but low in calories and fat, this superb appetizer is also ideal as a light lunch dish.

INGREDIENTS

Serves 6
6 zucchini
1 Spanish onion, very finely chopped
1 garlic clove, finely chopped
4–6 tablespoons well-seasoned French
   dressing
1 green bell pepper
3 tomatoes, peeled and seeded
1 tablespoon drained, rinsed capers
1 teaspoon chopped fresh parsley
1 teaspoon chopped fresh basil
sea salt and ground black pepper
parsley sprigs, to garnish

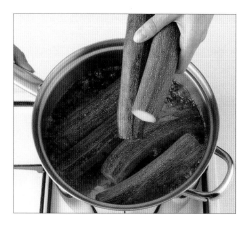

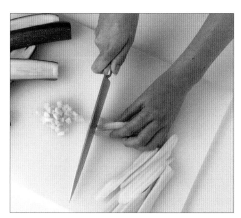

1 Trim the zucchini, but do not peel them. Bring a large, shallow pan of lightly salted water to a boil, add the zucchini and simmer for 2–3 minutes, until they are lightly cooked. Drain well.

2 Cut the zucchini in half lengthwise. Carefully scoop out the flesh, leaving the zucchini shells intact, and chop the flesh into small cubes. Place in a bowl and cover with half the chopped onion. Sprinkle with the chopped garlic. Drizzle 2 tablespoons of the dressing on top, cover and marinate for 2–3 hours. Wrap the zucchini shells tightly in plastic wrap, and chill them until they are required.

3 Cut the bell pepper in half and remove the core and seeds. Dice the flesh. Chop the tomatoes and capers finely. Stir the bell pepper, tomatoes and capers into the zucchini mixture with the remaining onion and the chopped herbs. Season with salt and pepper. Pour in enough of the remaining dressing to moisten the mixture and toss well. Spoon the filling into the zucchini shells, arrange on a platter and serve garnished with parsley.

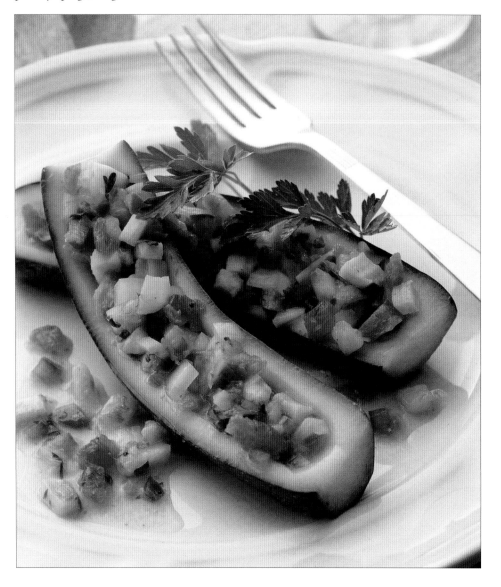

NUTRITION NOTES	
Per portion:	
Calories	95
Fat, total	7.3g
saturated fat	1.1g
polyunsaturated fat	0.9g
monounsaturated fat	4.9g
Carbohydrate	5.3g
sugar, total	4.75g
starch	0.2g
Fiber – NSP	1.95g
Sodium	60mg

Persian Omelet

Serve this spiced omelet hot or cold in wedges as an appetizer, or cut it into bite-size pieces for serving with drinks. The herbs and nuts add texture and taste.

INGREDIENTS

Serves 8

2 tablespoons olive oil or sunflower oil
2 leeks, finely chopped
12 ounces fresh spinach, washed and chopped, or 5 ounces thawed frozen chopped spinach, squeezed dry
12 eggs
8 scallions, finely chopped
2 handfuls fresh parsley, finely chopped
1–2 handfuls fresh cilantro, chopped
2 fresh tarragon sprigs, chopped, or ½ teaspoon dried tarragon
handful of fresh chives, chopped
1 small fresh dill sprig, chopped, or ¼ teaspoon dried dill
2–4 fresh mint sprigs, chopped
⅓ cup (1 ounce) walnuts or pecans, chopped
½ cup (1½ ounces) pine nuts
sea salt and ground black pepper
salad, to serve

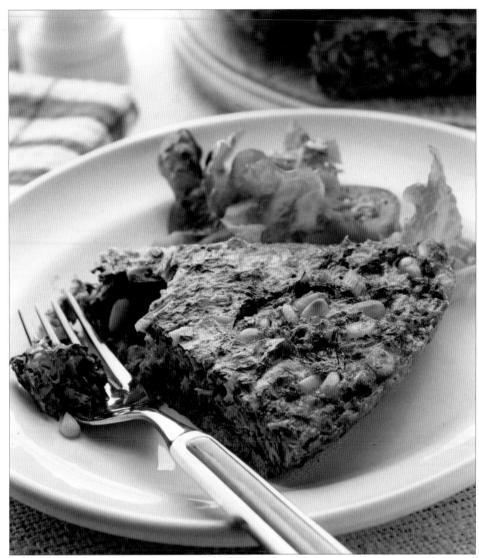

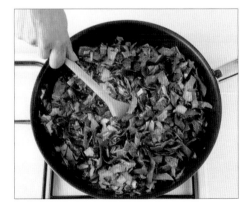

1 Heat the oil in a large, shallow pan that can be used under the broiler. Add the leeks and fry them gently for about 5 minutes, until they are just beginning to soften.

2 If using fresh spinach, add it to the pan containing the leeks and cook for 2–3 minutes over medium heat, until the spinach has just wilted.

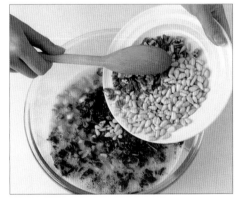

3 Beat the eggs in a bowl with a fork. Add the leek and spinach mixture (or the leeks with the thawed frozen spinach), then stir in the scallions, with all the herbs and nuts. Season with salt and pepper. Pour the mixture into the pan and cover with a lid or foil.

4 Cook over very gentle heat for 25 minutes, or until set. Remove the lid and brown the top under a hot broiler. Serve with salad.

NUTRITION NOTES	
Per portion:	
Calories	258
Fat, total	21g
saturated fat	3.9g
polyunsaturated fat	6.1g
monounsaturated fat	8.7g
Carbohydrate	2.8g
sugar, total	2.3g
starch	0.15g
Fiber – NSP	1.9g
Sodium	192mg

Eggplant and Smoked Trout Pâté

INGREDIENTS

Serves 6

1 large eggplant
2–3 garlic cloves, unpeeled
4 smoked trout fillets
juice of 1 lemon
sea salt and ground black pepper
toast triangles, to serve

--- NUTRITION NOTES ---

Per portion:	
Calories	145
Fat, total	4.7g
saturated fat	1.05g
polyunsaturated fat	1.6g
monounsaturated fat	1.6g
Carbohydrate	1.6g
sugar, total	1.1g
starch	0.5g
Fiber – NSP	1.1g
Sodium	89mg

1 Slice the eggplant thickly and spread out the slices in a steamer. Tuck the whole garlic cloves among the slices. Cover and steam over boiling water for 10–15 minutes, until both the eggplant slices and the garlic cloves are quite soft.

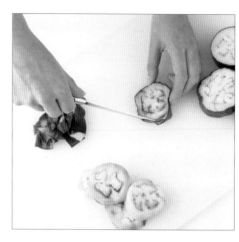

2 Carefully cut away and discard the skin from around the eggplant slices using a small, sharp knife.

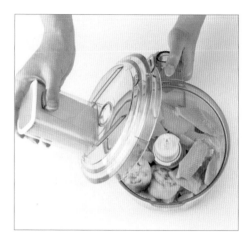

3 Skin the trout fillets and chop them roughly. Put them in a food processor. Squeeze the garlic flesh out of the skins and add it to the processor with the eggplant slices. Add the lemon juice and process until smooth. Spoon into a bowl and season. Cool, then chill. Serve with toast triangles.

Avocado and Strawberry Salad

The combination of avocado and strawberries works surprisingly well in this refreshing salad.

INGREDIENTS

Serves 6

2 large, ripe avocados
juice of 1–2 lemons
15 strawberries
½ cup low-fat plain yogurt
1–2 tablespoons chopped fresh mint
sea salt and ground black pepper
sprig of mint, to garnish

--- COOK'S TIP ---

Serve the salad right away, before the avocado slices have a chance to discolor.

1 Cut the avocados lengthwise in half and remove the skin and pits. Cut the avocado flesh into thin slices, then place the slices in a bowl and sprinkle with the lemon juice.

--- NUTRITION NOTES ---

Per portion:	
Calories	93
Fat, total	8g
saturated fat	1.75g
polyunsaturated fat	0.9g
monounsaturated fat	4.9g
Carbohydrate	3.5g
sugar, total	2.8g
starch	0g
Fiber – NSP	1.5g
Sodium	20mg

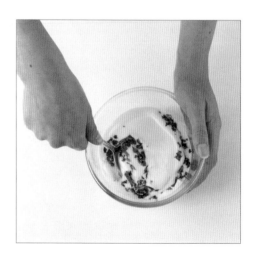

2 Halve or slice the strawberries and toss them lightly with the avocado slices in the bowl. Mix the yogurt with enough cold water to give a pouring consistency. Stir in the chopped mint and season. Spoon the dressing over the salad, garnish with mint and serve.

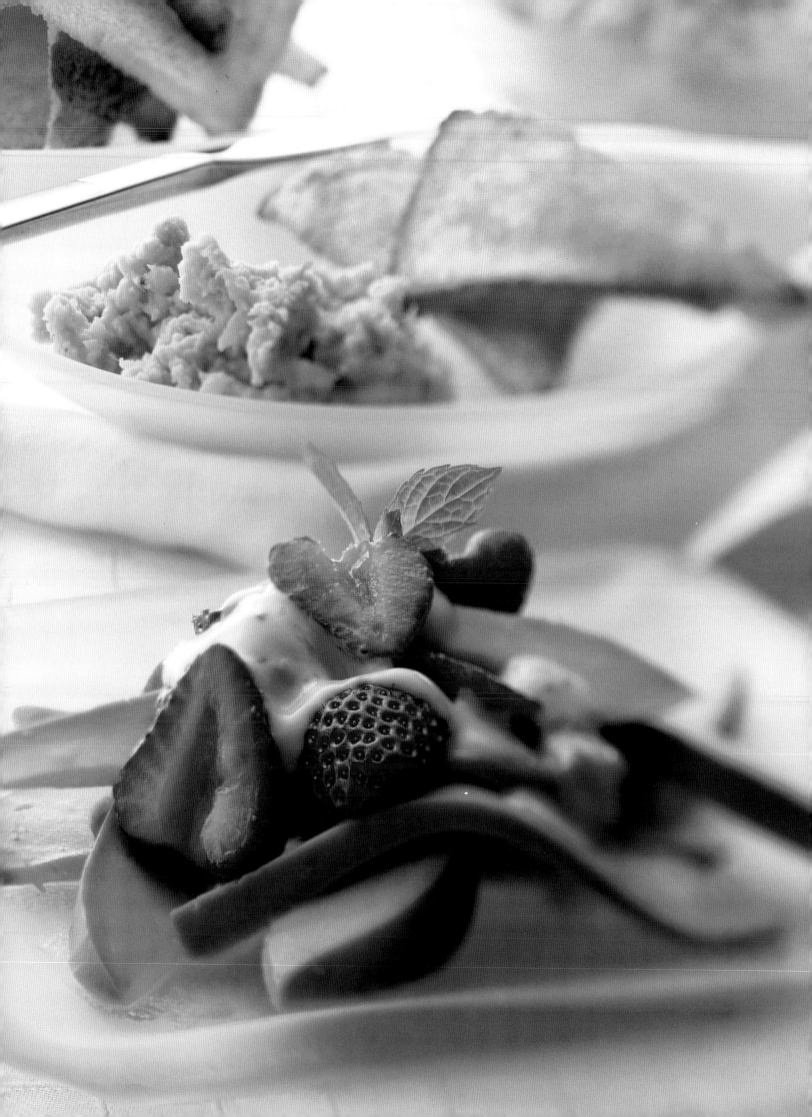

Sweet Potato and Red Pepper Soup

As colorful as it is good to eat, this soup is a sure winner.

INGREDIENTS

Serves 6

1¼ pounds sweet potatoes
2 red bell peppers, about 8 ounces,
   seeded and cubed
1 onion, roughly chopped
2 large garlic cloves, roughly chopped
1¼ cups dry white wine
5 cups vegetable or chicken broth
sea salt and ground black pepper
Tabasco sauce (optional)
country bread, to serve

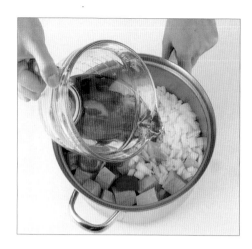

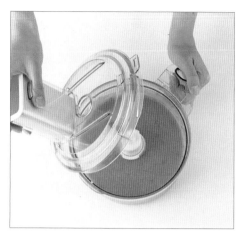

1 Peel the sweet potatoes and cut them into cubes. Put the cubes in a large saucepan with the red peppers, onion, garlic, wine and vegetable or chicken broth. Bring to a boil, lower the heat and simmer for 30 minutes, or until all the vegetables are quite soft.

2 Transfer the mixture to a food processor or blender and process until smooth. Season to taste with salt, pepper and a generous dash of Tabasco, if desired. Pour into a tureen or serving bowl and let cool slightly. Serve warm or at room temperature, with bread.

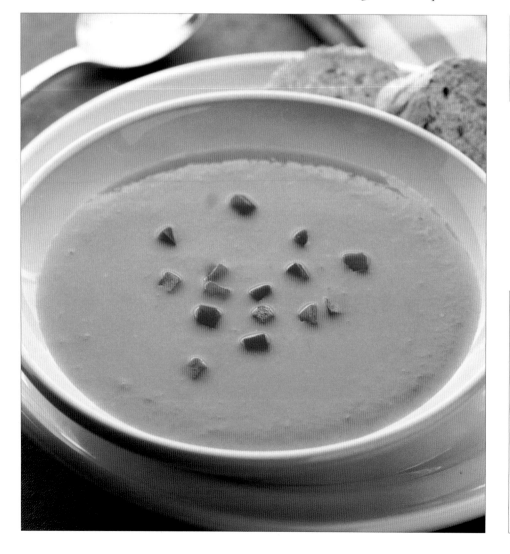

COOK'S TIP

Garnish the soup with finely diced red, green or yellow bell pepper, if you like.

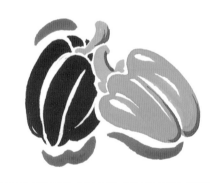

NUTRITION NOTES

Per portion:

Calories	122
Fat, total	0.4g
saturated fat	0.1g
polyunsaturated fat	0.17g
monounsaturated fat	0g
Carbohydrate	21.4g
sugar, total	7.9g
starch	13.2g
Fiber – NSP	2.8g
Sodium	37mg

Garlic Lentil Soup

High in fiber, lentils make a very tasty soup. Unlike many legumes, they do not need to be soaked before being cooked.

INGREDIENTS

Serves 6

1 cup (8 ounces) red lentils, rinsed
   and drained
2 onions, finely chopped
2 large garlic cloves, finely chopped
1 carrot, very finely chopped
2 tablespoons olive oil
2 bay leaves
generous pinch of dried marjoram
   or oregano
6¼ cups vegetable broth
2 tablespoons red wine vinegar
sea salt and ground black pepper
celery leaves, to garnish
crusty rolls, to serve

COOK'S TIP

If you buy your lentils loose, remember to pour them into a sieve or colander and pick them over, removing any pieces of grit, before rinsing them.

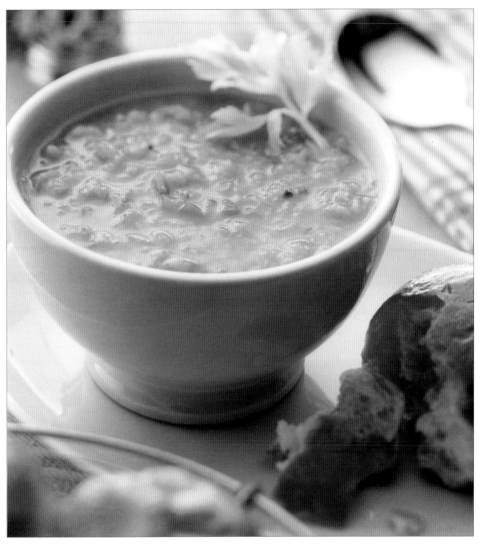

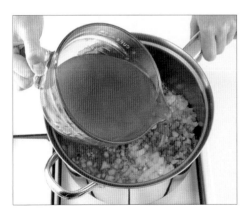

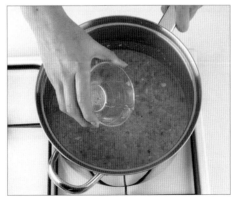

1 Put all the ingredients except the vinegar, seasoning and garnish in a large, heavy saucepan. Bring to a boil over medium heat, then lower the heat and simmer for 1½ hours, stirring the soup occasionally to prevent the lentils from sticking to the bottom of the pan.

2 Remove the bay leaves and add the red wine vinegar, with salt and pepper to taste. If the soup is too thick, thin it with a little extra vegetable broth or water. Serve the soup in heated bowls, garnished with celery leaves and accompanied by crusty rolls.

NUTRITION NOTES

Per portion:	
Calories	167
Fat, total	5.6g
saturated fat	0.8g
polyunsaturated fat	0.65g
monounsaturated fat	3.7g
Carbohydrate	23.6g
sugar, total	2.6g
starch	19.3g
Fiber – NSP	2.45g
Sodium	18.5mg

Green Pea Soup with Spinach

This lovely green soup would also make a nice lunch, served with crusty whole-wheat bread or a dinner served with a turkey or cheese sandwich.

INGREDIENTS

Serves 6
generous 3 cups shelled fresh or
   frozen peas
1 leek, finely sliced
2 garlic cloves, crushed
2 Canadian bacon slices,
   finely diced
5 cups ham or chicken broth
2 tablespoons olive oil
2 ounces fresh spinach, shredded
1½ ounces green cabbage, very
   finely shredded
½ small iceberg lettuce, very finely
   shredded
1 celery stalk, finely chopped
1 cup watercress, finely chopped
large handful of parsley, finely chopped
4 teaspoons chopped fresh mint
pinch of ground mace
sea salt and ground black pepper

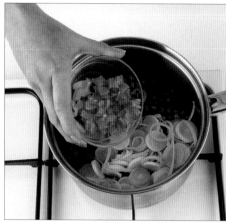

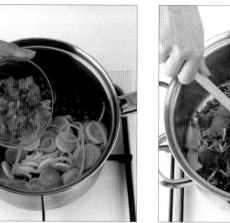

1 Put the peas, leek, garlic and bacon in a large saucepan. Add the broth, bring to a boil, then lower the heat and simmer for 20 minutes.

2 About 5 minutes before the pea mixture is ready, heat the oil in a large deep frying pan.

— COOK'S TIP —

Use 1 ounce frozen leaf spinach if fresh spinach is not available.

3 Add the spinach, cabbage, lettuce, celery, watercress and herbs. Cover and cook over low heat until soft.

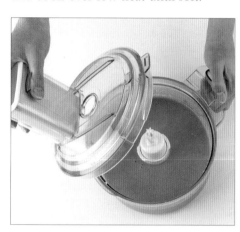

4 Transfer the pea mixture to a food processor or blender; process until smooth. Return to the saucepan, add the softened vegetables and herbs and heat through. Season with mace, salt and pepper and serve.

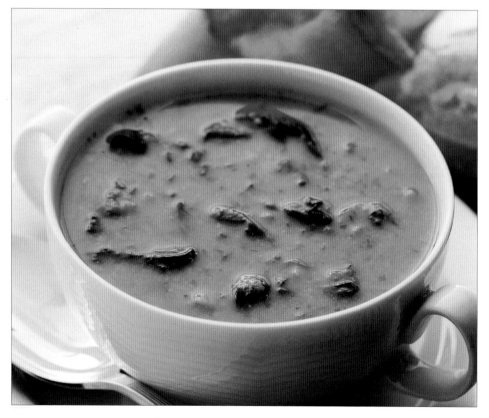

— NUTRITION NOTES —

Per portion:	
Calories	140
Fat, total	7.6g
saturated fat	1.45g
polyunsaturated fat	1.2g
monounsaturated fat	4.4g
Carbohydrate	10g
sugar, total	2.7g
starch	5.8g
Fiber – NSP	4.4g
Sodium	165mg

Cream of Celery Root and Spinach Soup

Celery root has a wonderful flavor that is reminiscent of celery but also adds a slightly nutty taste. Here it is combined with spinach to make a delicious soup.

INGREDIENTS

Serves 6

1 leek
1¼ pounds celery root
4 cups water
1 cup dry white wine
7 ounces fresh spinach leaves
sea salt, ground black pepper and
   grated nutmeg
skim milk (optional)
⅓ cup (1 ounce) pine nuts

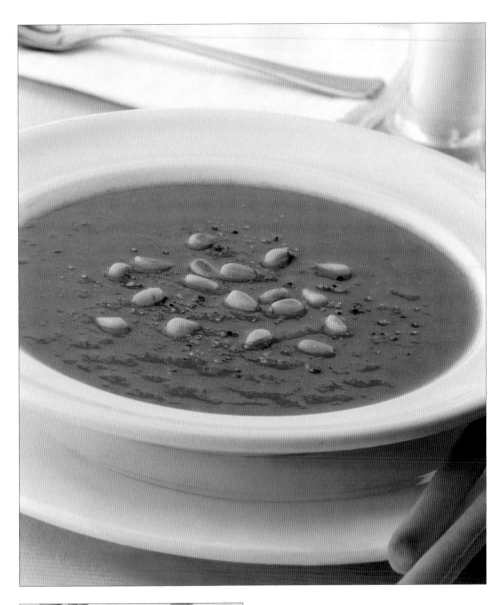

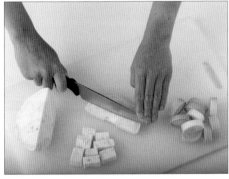

1 Trim and slit the leek. Rinse it under running water to remove any grit, then slice it thickly. Peel the celery root and dice the flesh.

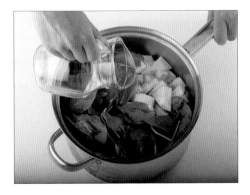

2 Mix the water and wine in a pitcher. Place the leek, celery root and spinach in a deep saucepan and pour the liquid over them. Bring to a boil, lower the heat and simmer for 10–15 minutes, until the vegetables are soft.

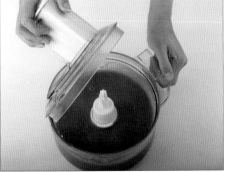

3 Purée the vegetable mixture, in batches if necessary, in a food processor or blender. Return to the clean pan and season to taste with salt, pepper and nutmeg. If the soup is too thick, thin it with a little water or skim milk. Reheat gently.

4 Sauté the pine nuts in a dry nonstick frying pan until golden. Sprinkle them over the soup and serve.

NUTRITION NOTES	
Per portion:	
Calories	82
Fat, total	3.5g
saturated fat	0.25g
polyunsaturated fat	1.9g
monounsaturated fat	0.85g
Carbohydrate	3.25g
sugar, total	2.7g
starch	0.5g
Fiber – NSP	4g
Sodium	124mg

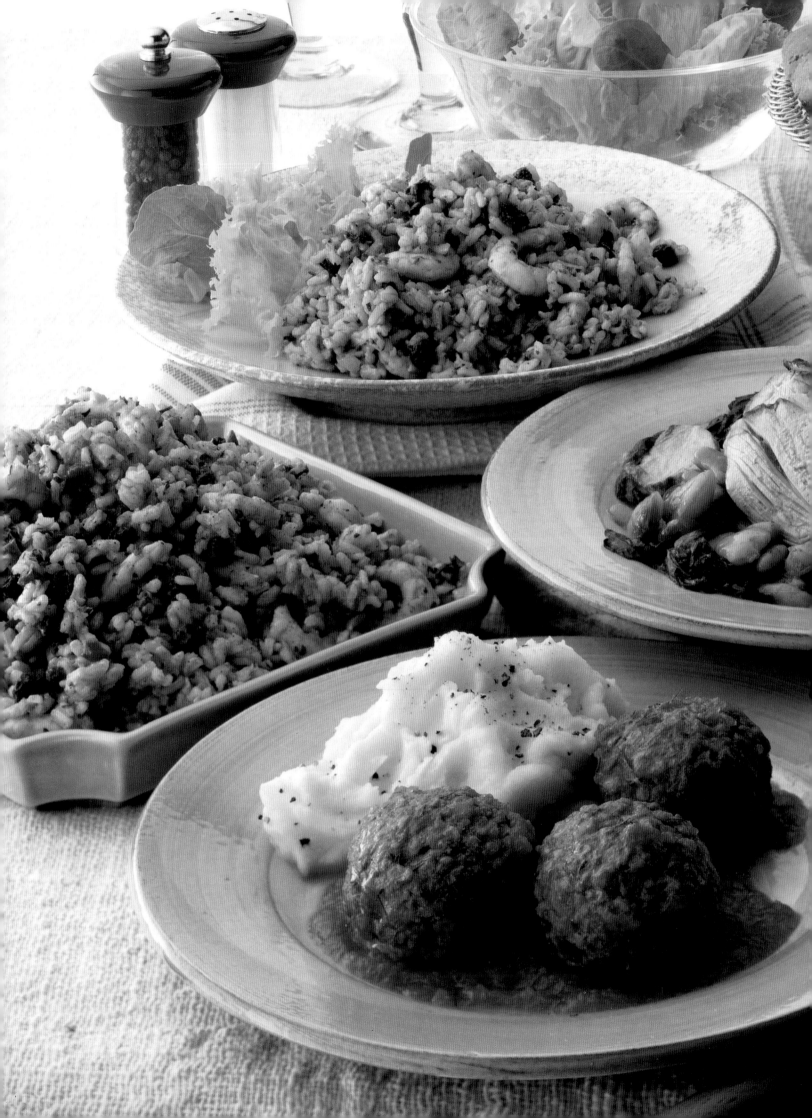

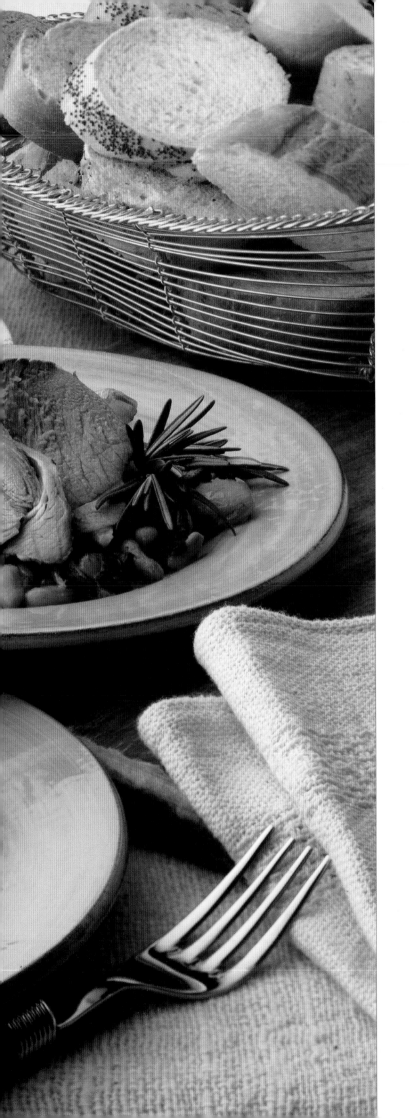

FISH, MEAT AND POULTRY

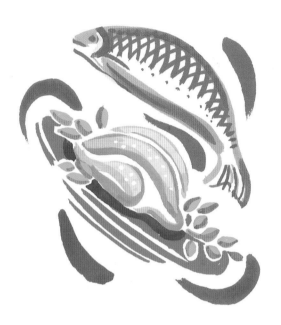

Fish is an excellent food for diabetics, and such dishes as pilaf with spicy shrimp and parcels of filo pastry filled with sardines are both healthy and light. Meat dishes tend to be heartier fare, but they need to be high in fiber for diabetics. The selection here includes beef and lentil balls cooked in a tomato sauce, leg of lamb roasted until tender with cannellini beans and green peppercorns, and sausages combined with mixed beans and bacon to make a warming casserole.

Fennel and Smoked Haddock Chowder

This soup is substantial enough to serve as a main meal with plenty of poppy seed bread.

INGREDIENTS

Serves 8
1 large fennel bulb
2 large leeks, very finely sliced
8 ounces new potatoes, scrubbed,
   halved or quartered if large
1 teaspoon dill seed
2 large garlic cloves, thinly sliced
½ lemon
6¼ cups water
1¼ cups dry white wine
ground black pepper
8 ounces smoked haddock fillet,
   skinned
sea salt
chopped fresh parsley, to garnish

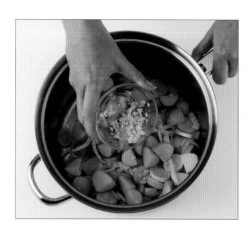

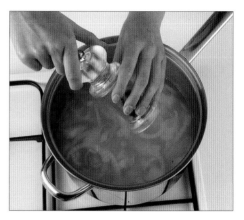

1 Quarter the fennel, cut away the core and slice each piece very finely. Place in a large saucepan with the leeks, potatoes, dill seed and garlic. Cut the lemon half into thick slices and add these to the pan. Pour the water and wine into the pan.

2 Season with plenty of ground black pepper, then bring to a boil, lower the heat and simmer for about 30 minutes, or until the potatoes and fennel are both quite soft.

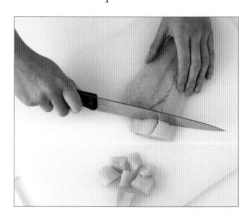

3 Cut the haddock into chunks, add to the pan and simmer the mixture for 10 minutes more. Remove the lemon slices. Stir the soup gently. Add salt and pepper to taste. Sprinkle with parsley and serve.

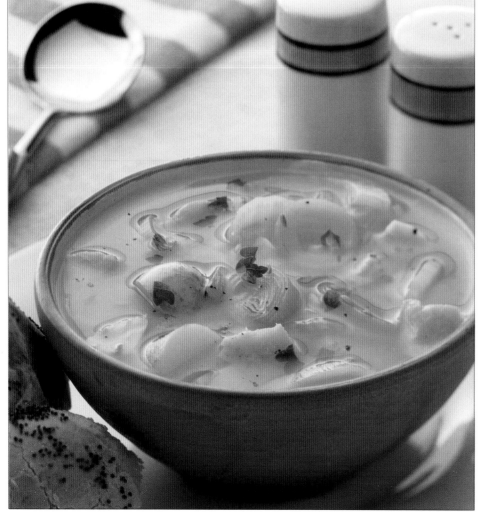

— NUTRITION NOTES —	
Per portion:	
Calories	75
Fat, total	0.5g
saturated fat	0.1g
polyunsaturated fat	0.15g
monounsaturated fat	0.1g
Carbohydrate	6g
sugar, total	1.5g
starch	4.35g
Fiber – NSP	1.2g
Sodium	221mg

Spaghetti with Smoked Salmon

INGREDIENTS

Serves 6

2 tablespoons olive oil
4 ounces button mushrooms, finely
  sliced (1 cup)
1 cup dry white wine
1½ teaspoons chopped fresh dill or
  1 teaspoon dried dill
handful of fresh chives, snipped
1¼ cups very low-fat unsweetened soy
  cream or very low-fat fromage frais
8 ounces smoked salmon, cut into
  thin strips
ground black pepper
lemon juice
12 ounces fresh spaghetti or linguine
chives, to garnish

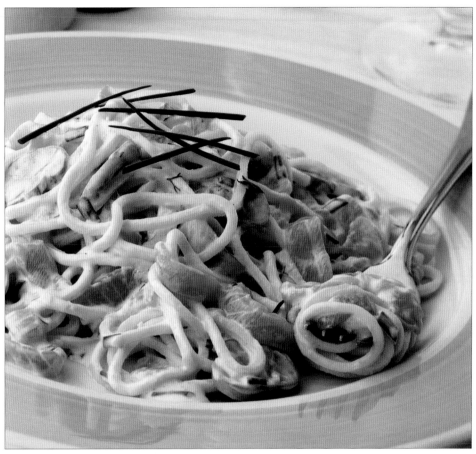

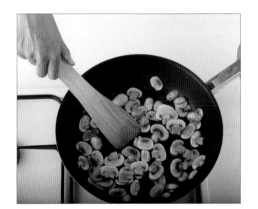

1 Heat the oil in a large nonstick
frying pan. Add the finely sliced
mushrooms and fry them over gentle
heat for 4–5 minutes, until they are
softened but not colored.

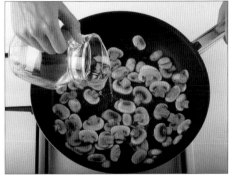

2 Pour the white wine into the pan.
Increase the heat and boil rapidly
for about 5 minutes, until the wine has
reduced considerably.

—— COOK'S TIP ——

Soy cream may be an acquired taste, but it
is a very successful low-fat substitute for
dairy cream in dishes like this one, with a
strong flavor of their own.

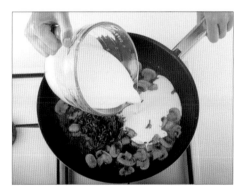

3 Stir in the herbs and the soy cream
or fromage frais. Fold in the salmon
and reheat gently, but do not let the
sauce boil or it will curdle. Stir in
pepper and lemon juice to taste. Cover
the pan and keep the sauce warm.

4 Cook the pasta in a large saucepan
of lightly salted boiling water until
just tender. Drain, rinse thoroughly in
boiling water and drain again. Turn
into a warmed serving dish and toss
gently with the salmon sauce before
serving, garnished with chives.

—— NUTRITION NOTES ——

Per portion:

Calories	346
Fat, total	8.3g
saturated fat	1.35g
polyunsaturated fat	1.6g
monounsaturated fat	4.5g
Carbohydrate	42.4g
sugar, total	5.8g
starch	36.5g
Fiber – NSP	5.16g
Sodium	800mg

Sardine and Spinach Parcels

If you need encouragement to eat more oily fish, this recipe will provide the perfect excuse.

INGREDIENTS

Serves 6

2 x 4¼-ounce cans large sardines in oil
3 leeks, finely chopped
11 ounces fresh spinach leaves, finely shredded
2 tomatoes, peeled, seeded and finely chopped
sea salt and ground black pepper
lemon juice
24 sheets of filo pastry, about 8 inches square, thawed if frozen
2 tablespoons olive oil, for brushing filo
salad leaves, to garnish

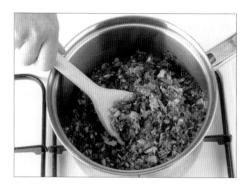

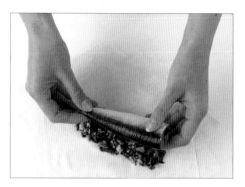

1 Preheat the oven to 350°F. Drain the oil from one of the cans of sardines into a large saucepan. Set 6 sardines aside. Heat the oil and fry the leeks for 5 minutes. Add the spinach and tomatoes and cook over low heat for 5 minutes, until soft. Add salt, pepper and lemon juice to taste.

2 Stack 4 sheets of filo, lightly brushing each sheet with olive oil and laying it at an angle of 45 degrees to the one below. Spoon one-sixth of the vegetable mixture across the center of the top sheet. Press a sardine into the middle of the vegetable mixture.

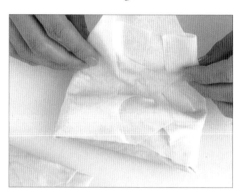

3 Fold over the filo to make a parcel, lightly brushing each fold with olive oil. Brush the top of the parcel with oil and place it on a baking sheet. Make 5 more parcels. Bake the parcels for 20 minutes, or until the filo is crisp and brown. Garnish with salad leaves.

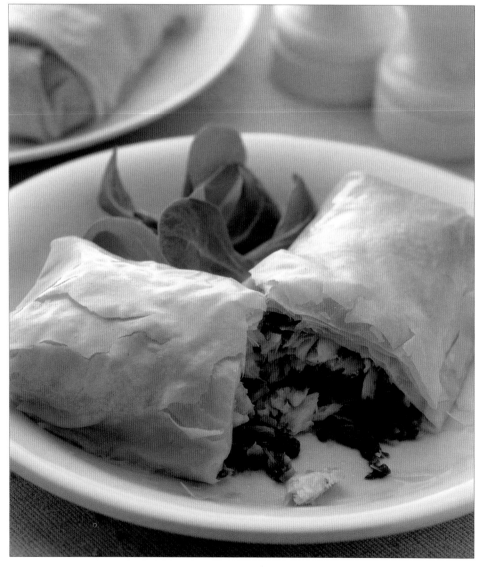

— NUTRITION NOTES —	
Per portion:	
Calories	251
Fat, total	12g
saturated fat	1.9g
polyunsaturated fat	2.8g
monounsaturated fat	5.65g
Carbohydrate	22.5g
sugar, total	2.5g
starch	20g
Fiber – NSP	2.2g
Sodium	253mg

Turkish Shrimp Pilaf

INGREDIENTS

Serves 6

4 tablespoons olive oil
1 onion, finely chopped
2 large red bell peppers, seeded and
  finely chopped
2 garlic cloves, finely chopped
1½ cups (12 ounces) raw brown rice
1 teaspoon ground allspice
1 teaspoon ground cumin
2 teaspoons dried mint or basil
8 ounces cooked peeled shrimp,
  thawed if frozen
3 tablespoons currants
sea salt and ground black pepper
juice of 2 large lemons
2 handfuls fresh parsley, finely chopped
salad, to serve

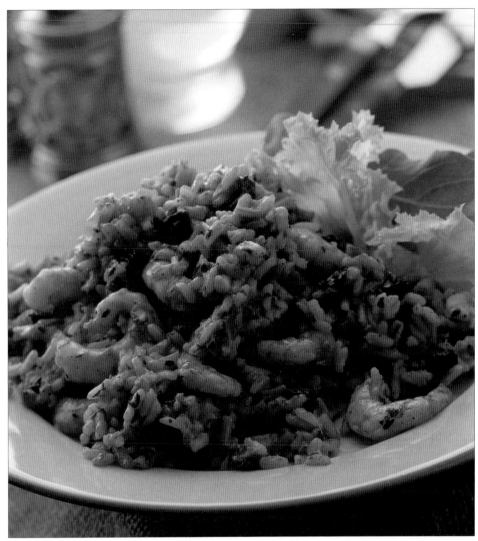

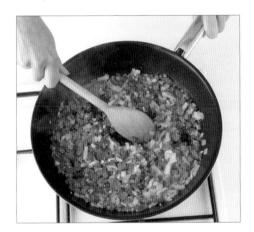

1 Heat the oil in a large nonstick frying pan. Fry the onion, peppers and garlic over low heat for 10 minutes, until softened but not browned.

— NUTRITION NOTES —

Per portion:	
Calories	383
Fat, total	12.6g
saturated fat	2g
polyunsaturated fat	1.7g
monounsaturated fat	7.9g
Carbohydrate	58g
sugar, total	10g
starch	47g
Fiber – NSP	2.4g
Sodium	606mg

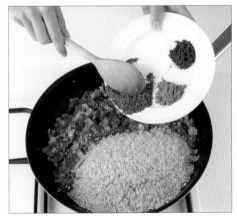

2 Add the rice, spices and mint or basil. Stir over the heat for 2–3 minutes, then add enough water to cover the rice. Bring to a boil, lower the heat and simmer, uncovered, for 10–15 minutes, or until the rice is just tender, but still has a little bite to it.

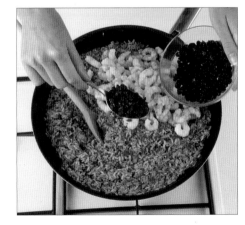

3 Add the shrimp, currants and a little salt and pepper to taste. Cook for about 4 minutes more, until the shrimp are heated through, then add the lemon juice and chopped parsley. Serve the pilaf warm or cold, with salad.

Spiced Round of Beef

A spicy marinade gives the beef a wonderful flavor, while slow cooking keeps it very moist.

INGREDIENTS

Serves 8

2 teaspoons coriander seeds
1 teaspoon each aniseed, fennel seeds, dried thyme, ground cloves, sea salt and ground black pepper
1/2 teaspoon ground cinnamon
2 1/2 cups dry white wine
2 1/4–2 1/2-pound round of beef
2 tablespoons olive oil
2 onions, finely chopped
2 carrots, finely chopped
2 celery stalks, finely chopped
1 parsnip, finely chopped
4 green beans, finely chopped
8 mushrooms, finely chopped
1 1/4 cups beef or chicken broth, preferably homemade
7 tablespoons dry red wine
2 fresh parsley sprigs
baked potatoes, to serve

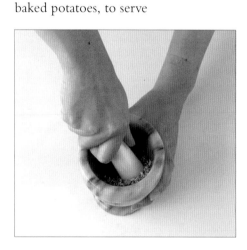

1 Put the coriander seeds in a mortar and pound them with a pestle. Stir in the rest of the spices and seasonings, then pour the mixture into a bowl and stir in the white wine.

COOK'S TIP

Patience is the secret of this superb casserole. Marinate the meat for the time stated, and cook it very slowly.

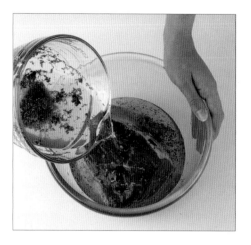

2 Put the beef in a deep glass or ceramic bowl. Pour the marinade over the beef, cover the bowl and let marinate in the refrigerator for about 24 hours. Turn the beef occasionally.

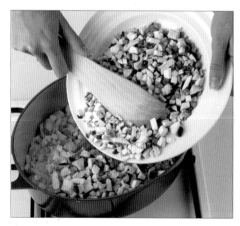

3 Preheat the oven to 300°F. Heat the oil in a deep casserole just large enough to hold the beef snugly. Add all the vegetables and cook over gentle heat for 15–20 minutes, or until they start to soften.

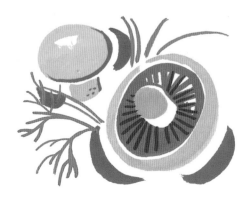

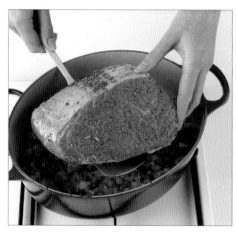

4 Lift the beef out of the marinade and place on top of the vegetables. Strain 1 1/4 cups of the marinade into a measuring cup and add the broth and red wine.

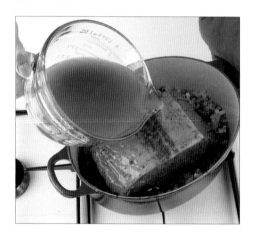

5 Pour the liquid over the beef. Add the parsley, cover and place in the oven. Bake for 2–3 hours, or until the beef is tender. Serve with potatoes.

--- NUTRITION NOTES ---

Per portion:

Calories	260
Fat, total	7.95g
saturated fat	2g
polyunsaturated fat	0.73g
monounsaturated fat	4.25g
Carbohydrate	4.3g
sugar, total	2.8g
starch	0.8g
Fiber – NSP	1.25g
Sodium	203mg

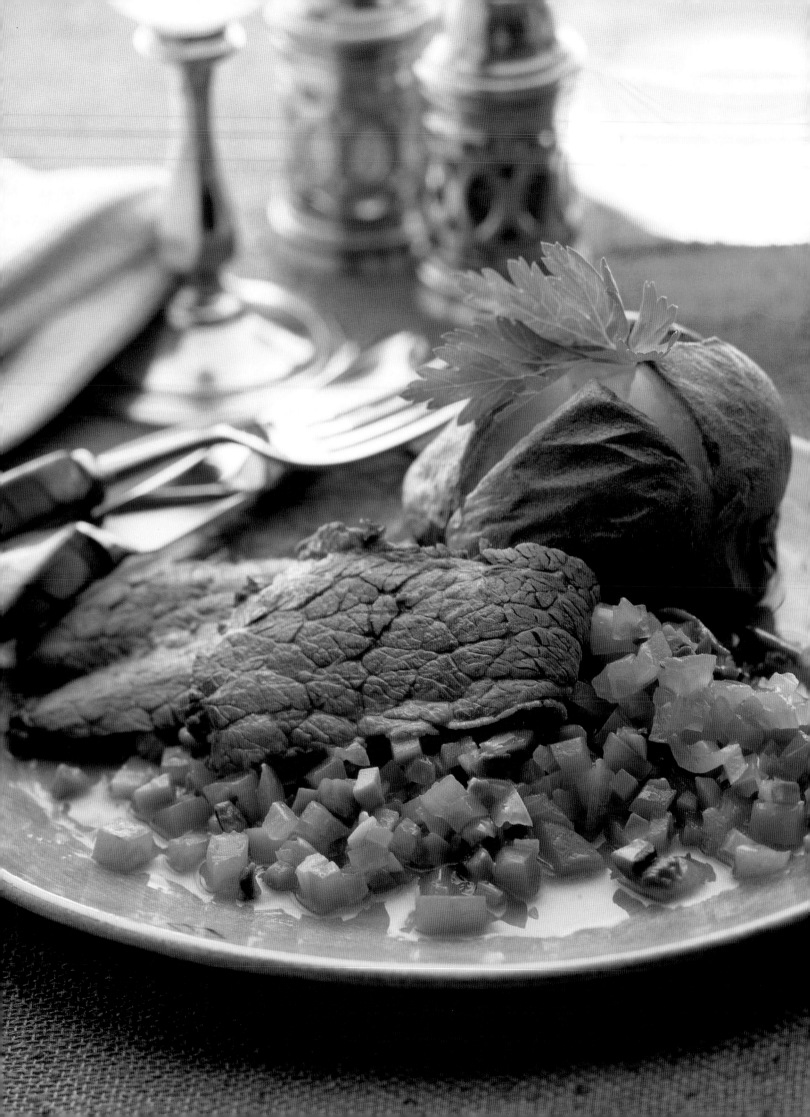

Lamb with Beans and Green Peppercorns

Roasting the lamb slowly on a bed of beans results in a dish that combines meltingly tender meat with plenty of soluble fiber.

INGREDIENTS

Serves 6

8–10 garlic cloves, peeled
4–4½-pound leg of lamb
2 tablespoons olive oil
14 ounces fresh spinach leaves
14-ounce can cannellini beans, drained
14-ounce can lima beans, drained
2 large fresh rosemary sprigs
1–2 tablespoons drained green
  peppercorns
potatoes, to serve

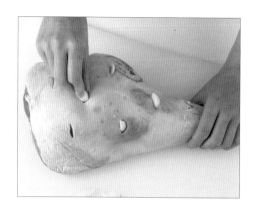

1 Preheat the oven to 300°F. Set 4 garlic cloves aside and slice the rest lengthwise into three or four pieces each. Make shallow slits in the skin of the lamb and insert a piece of garlic into each one.

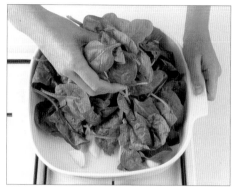

2 Heat the oil in a heavy flameproof casserole or roasting pan that is just large enough to hold the lamb. Add the reserved garlic and the spinach and cook briskly for 4–5 minutes, or until the spinach is wilted.

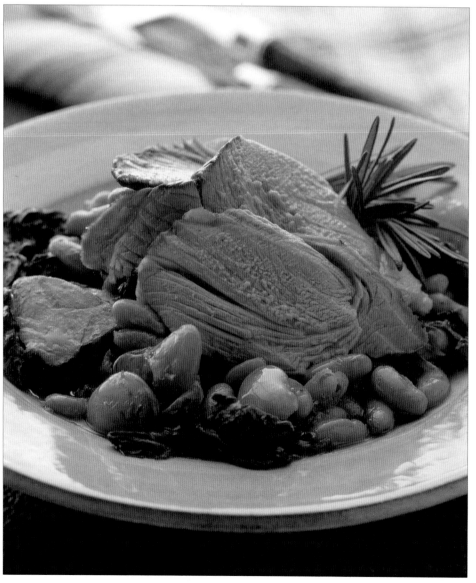

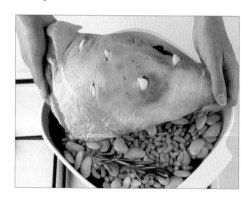

3 Add the beans and tuck the rosemary sprigs and peppercorns among them. Place the lamb on top. Cover with foil or a lid. Bake the lamb for 3–4 hours, until it is cooked to your taste. Serve with the spinach and beans and potatoes.

NUTRITION NOTES	
Per portion:	
Calories	312
Fat, total	14.5g
saturated fat	4.6g
polyunsaturated fat	1.4g
monounsaturated fat	6.9g
Carbohydrate	17.8g
sugar, total	2.3g
starch	14.2g
Fiber – NSP	6g
Sodium	172mg

Smoked Bacon, Sausage and Bean Casserole

This casserole is the perfect choice for a winter evening.

INGREDIENTS

Serves 6
⅔ cup each dried black-eyed peas and cannellini beans
1 tablespoon olive oil
6 slices smoked lean bacon
6 large country pork sausages
3 large carrots, halved
3 large onions, halved
1 small garlic bulb, separated into cloves
4 bay leaves
2 fresh thyme sprigs
1–2 tablespoons drained green peppercorns
1¼ cups unsalted vegetable broth or water
1¼ cups dry red wine
sea salt and ground black pepper
thyme sprigs, to garnish
green salad, to serve

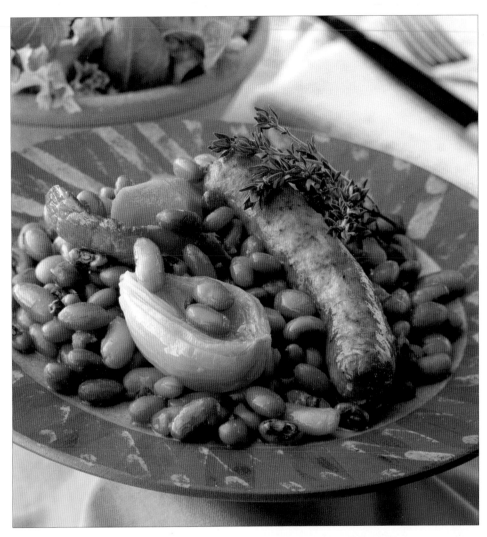

1 Bring a large saucepan of unsalted water to a boil. Add the beans and boil vigorously for 30 minutes. Drain and set aside.

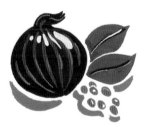

NUTRITION NOTES

Per portion:	
Calories	410
Fat, total	20.5g
saturated fat	6.7g
polyunsaturated fat	2.3g
monounsaturated fat	10.25g
Carbohydrate	33.8g
sugar, total	5.4g
starch	25.6g
Fiber – NSP	7g
Sodium	467mg

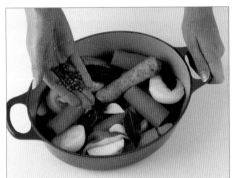

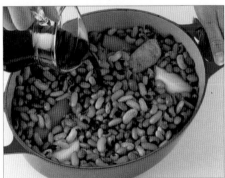

2 Pour the olive oil into a large, heavy flameproof casserole, then lay the bacon slices on top. Add the whole sausages and the halved carrots and onions. Peel but do not slice the garlic cloves, then press them into the mixture with the bay leaves, thyme sprigs and drained peppercorns. Spoon the cooked, drained beans over the top of the mixture.

3 Pour in the broth or water and wine. Cover the casserole and bring the liquid to a boil over medium heat. Reduce the heat to the lowest setting and simmer for 4–6 hours, stirring occasionally and topping up the liquid if necessary. Stir the mixture, remove the bay leaves and season before serving, garnished with thyme. Serve from the casserole, accompanied by a green salad.

Two-way Chicken with Vegetables

This tender, slow-cooked chicken makes a tasty lunch or supper, with the stock and remaining vegetables providing a nourishing soup as a second meal!

INGREDIENTS

Serves 6

3-pound chicken
2 onions, quartered
3 carrots, thickly sliced
2 celery stalks, chopped
1 parsnip or turnip, thickly sliced
½ cup button mushrooms, chopped
1–2 fresh thyme sprigs or 1 teaspoon
  dried thyme
4 bay leaves
large bunch of fresh parsley
new potatoes or pasta and sugar snap
  peas or green beans, to serve
1 cup whole-wheat pasta shapes
sea salt and ground black pepper
whole-wheat bread, to serve

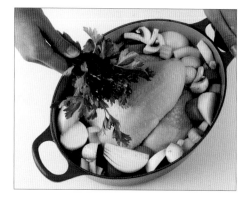

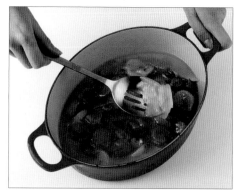

1 Trim the chicken of any excess fat. Put it in a flameproof casserole and add the vegetables and herbs. Pour in water to cover. Bring to a boil, skimming off any scum. When the water boils, lower the heat and simmer, covered, for 2–3 hours. Remove the chicken, carve the meat neatly, discarding the skin and bones, and return any small pieces to the pan. Serve the chicken with some of the vegetables from the pan, plus new potatoes or pasta and sugar snap peas or green beans, if you like.

2 Remove the bay leaves and any large pieces of parsley and thyme from the pan. Let the remaining mixture cool, then chill it overnight. The next day, lift off the fat that has solidified on the surface. Reheat the soup gently.

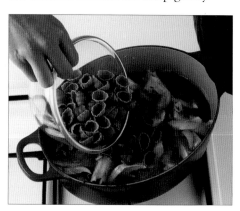

3 When the soup comes to a boil, add the pasta shapes, with salt, if needed, and cook for 10–12 minutes, or until the pasta is tender. Season with salt and pepper and garnish with parsley. Serve with whole-wheat bread.

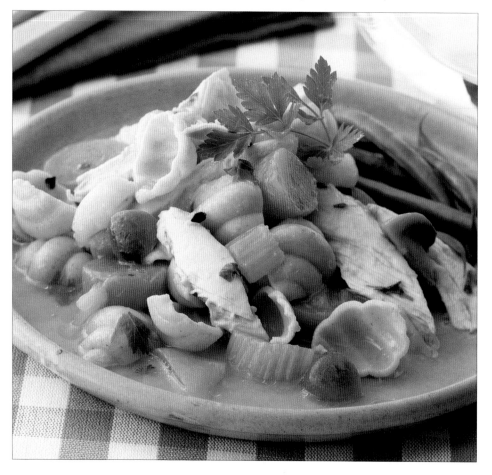

NUTRITION NOTES	
Per portion:	
Calories	212
Fat, total	3.3g
saturated fat	0.8g
polyunsaturated fat	0.8g
monounsaturated fat	1.3g
Carbohydrate	17.5g
sugar, total	3.7g
starch	12.7g
Fiber – NSP	3.15g
Sodium	130mg

Chicken Baked with Lima Beans and Garlic

A one-pot meal that combines chicken with leeks, fennel and garlic-flavored lima beans.

INGREDIENTS

Serves 6

2 leeks
1 small fennel bulb, roughly chopped
4 garlic cloves, peeled
Two 14-ounce cans lima
   beans, drained
2 large handfuls fresh parsley, chopped
1¼ cups dry white wine
1¼ cups vegetable broth
3-pound chicken
parsley sprigs, to garnish
cooked green vegetables, to serve

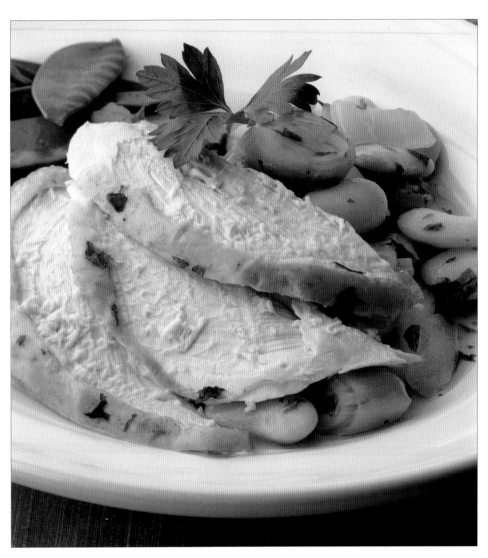

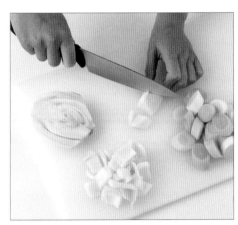

1 Preheat the oven to 350°F. Slit the leeks, wash out any grit, then slice them thickly. Cut the fennel into quarters, remove the core and chop the flesh roughly.

NUTRITION NOTES	
Per portion:	
Calories	304
Fat, total	3.4g
saturated fat	0.8g
polyunsaturated fat	0.9g
monounsaturated fat	1.2g
Carbohydrate	26.2g
sugar, total	3.2g
starch	21.2g
Fiber – NSP	8g
Sodium	105mg

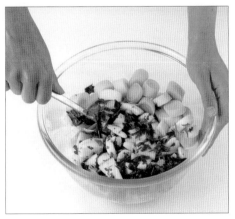

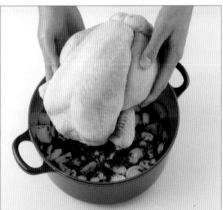

2 Mix the leeks, fennel, whole garlic cloves, limaw beans and chopped parsley in a bowl. Spread out the mixture on the bottom of a heavy flameproof casserole that is just large enough to hold the chicken. Pour in the white wine and vegetable broth.

3 Place the chicken on top. Bring to a boil, cover the casserole and transfer it to the oven. Bake for 1–1½ hours, until the chicken is cooked and so tender that it falls off the bone. Garnish with parsley and serve with lightly cooked green vegetables.

Beef and Lentil Balls with Tomato Sauce

Mixing lentils with the ground beef not only boosts the fiber content of these meatballs but also adds to the flavor.

INGREDIENTS

Serves 8
1 tablespoon olive oil
2 onions, finely chopped
2 celery stalks, finely chopped
2 large carrots, finely chopped
16 ounces lean ground beef
scant 1 cup (7 ounces) brown lentils
14-ounce can plum tomatoes
2 tablespoons tomato paste
2 bay leaves
1¼ cups vegetable broth
¾ cup dry red wine
2–3 tablespoons Worcestershire sauce
2 eggs
2 large handfuls of fresh
   parsley, chopped
sea salt and ground black pepper
mashed potatoes and green salad,
   to serve

For the tomato sauce
4 onions, finely chopped
Two 14-ounce cans plum tomatoes
4 tablespoons dry red wine
3 fresh dill sprigs, finely chopped

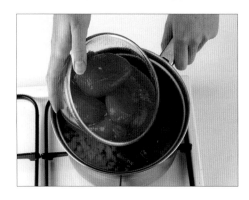

1 Start by making the tomato sauce. Combine the onions, canned plum tomatoes and red wine in a saucepan. Bring to a boil, lower the heat, cover the pan and simmer for 30 minutes. Purée the mixture in a blender or food processor, then return it to the saucepan and set it aside.

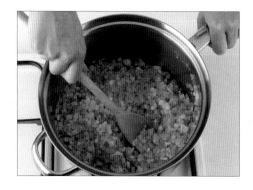

2 Make the meatballs. Heat the oil in a large, heavy saucepan and cook the chopped onions, celery and carrots for 5–10 minutes, or until the onions and carrots are softened but not browned.

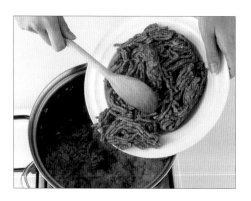

3 Add the ground beef and cook over high heat, stirring frequently, until the meat is lightly browned.

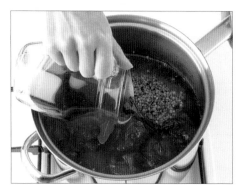

4 Add the lentils, tomatoes, tomato paste, bay leaves, vegetable broth and wine. Mix well and bring to a boil, breaking up the tomatoes with a spoon. Lower the heat and simmer for 20–30 minutes, until the liquid has been completely absorbed. Remove the bay leaves, then stir the Worcestershire sauce into the lentil mixture.

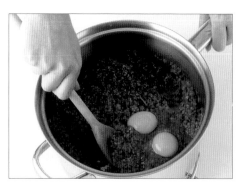

5 Remove the pan from the heat and add the eggs and parsley. Season with salt and pepper and mix well, then allow the mixture to cool. Meanwhile, preheat the oven to 350°F.

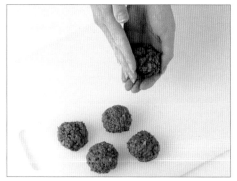

6 Shape the beef mixture into neat balls, rolling them in your hands. Arrange in an ovenproof dish and bake for 25 minutes. While the meatballs are baking, reheat the tomato sauce. Just before serving, stir in the chopped dill. Pour the tomato sauce over the meatballs and serve. Mashed potatoes and salad make excellent accompaniments.

NUTRITION NOTES	
Per portion:	
Calories	272
Fat, total	9.3g
saturated fat	2.9g
polyunsaturated fat	0.8g
monounsaturated fat	4.2g
Carbohydrate	22.65g
sugar, total	9g
starch	11.5g
Fiber – NSP	4.5g
Sodium	155mg

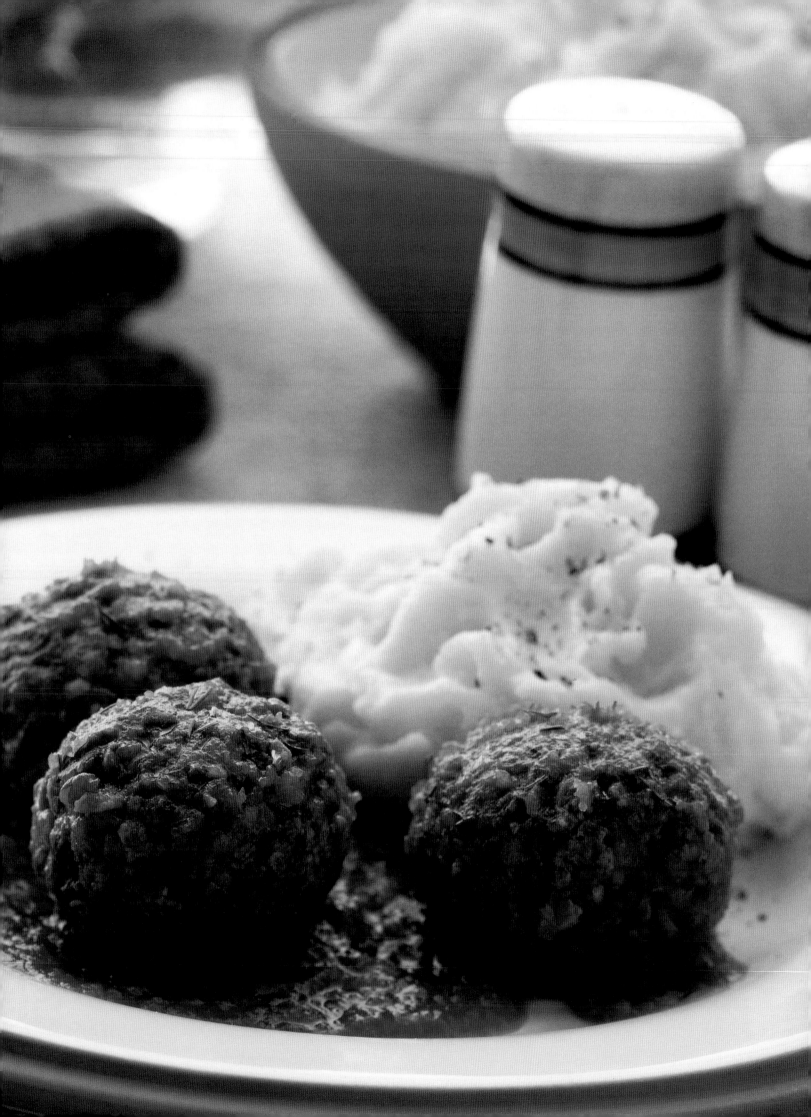

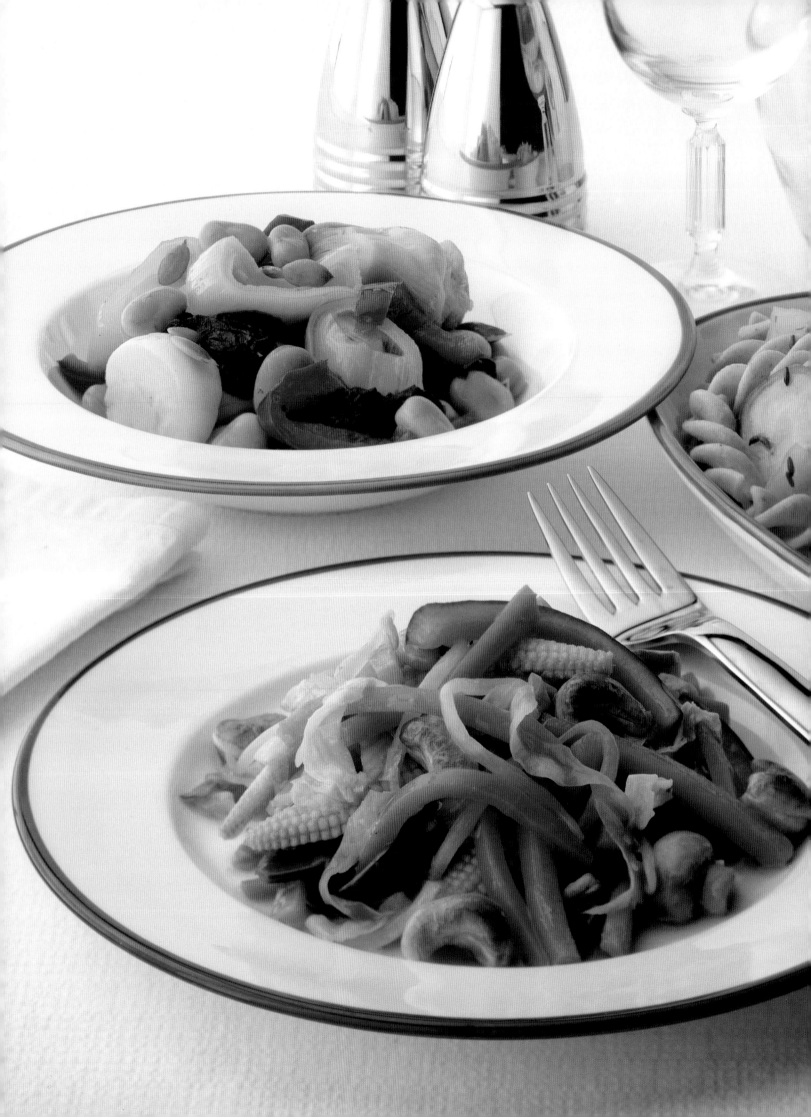

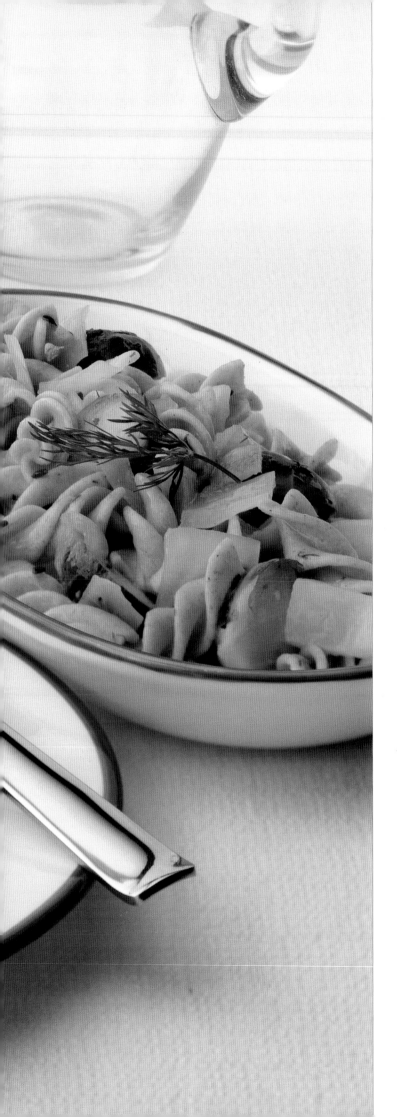

VEGETABLES AND VEGETARIAN DISHES

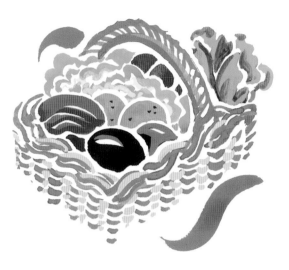

The increasing popularity of vegetarian food is good news for diabetics. Dishes such as a casserole of red cabbage and apple or baked vegetables with artichokes can be served as main meals, or in smaller portions as accompaniments to meat or fish dishes. Others, such as a risotto made with red peppers and a pie of mushrooms and sunflower seeds, make excellent meals on their own, with a salad or served with another vegetable.

Red Cabbage and Apple Casserole

The brilliant color and pungent flavor make this an excellent winter dish. Serve it solo, with plenty of rye bread, or as a vegetable side dish.

INGREDIENTS

Serves 6

3 onions, chopped
2 fennel bulbs, roughly chopped
1½ pounds red cabbage, shredded
2 tablespoons caraway seeds
3 large tart eating apples or 1 large
    cooking apple
6 slices Canadian bacon (optional)
1¼ cups low-fat plain yogurt
1 tablespoon creamed horseradish sauce
sea salt and ground black pepper

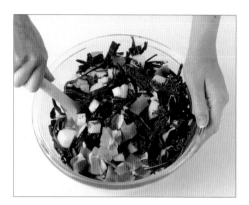

1 Preheat the oven to 300°F. Mix the onions, fennel, red cabbage and caraway seeds in a bowl. Peel, core and chop the apples and chop the bacon slices, if using, then stir them into the cabbage mixture. Transfer to a casserole. Mix the yogurt with the creamed horseradish sauce.

2 Stir the yogurt and horseradish mixture into the casserole, season with salt and pepper and cover tightly. Bake for 1½ hours, stirring once or twice. Serve hot.

NUTRITION NOTES	
Per portion:	
Calories	158
Fat, total	9.7g
saturated fat	3.4g
polyunsaturated fat	1.4g
monounsaturated fat	4.05g
Carbohydrate	12.8g
sugar, total	11.6g
starch	0.2g
Fiber – NSP	4g
Sodium	378mg

Mixed Vegetables with Artichokes

Baking a vegetable medley in the oven is a wonderfully easy way of producing a quick and simple, wholesome midweek meal.

INGREDIENTS

Serves 4

2 tablespoons olive oil
1½ pounds frozen lima beans
4 turnips, peeled and sliced
4 leeks, sliced
1 red bell pepper, seeded and sliced
7 ounces fresh spinach leaves or
    4 ounces thawed frozen spinach,
    squeezed dry
Two 14-ounce cans artichoke hearts,
    drained
4 tablespoons pumpkin seeds
soy sauce
ground black pepper
rice, baked potatoes or whole-wheat
    bread, to serve

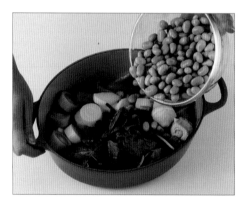

1 Preheat the oven to 350°F. Pour the oil into a casserole. Cook the lima beans in a saucepan of lightly salted boiling water for about 5 minutes. Drain the beans and place them with the turnips, leeks, red pepper slices, spinach and canned artichoke hearts in the casserole.

2 Cover the casserole and bake the vegetables for 30–40 minutes, or until the turnips are soft.

3 Stir in the pumpkin seeds and soy sauce to taste. Season with ground black pepper. Serve solo or with rice sprinkled with chopped fresh herbs, baked potatoes or bread.

NUTRITION NOTES	
Per portion:	
Calories	335
Fat, total	13.4g
saturated fat	2.2g
polyunsaturated fat	3.3g
monounsaturated fats	6.5g
Carbohydrate	34.95g
sugar, total	11.4g
starch	19.4g
Fiber – NSP	16.3g
Sodium	151.5mg

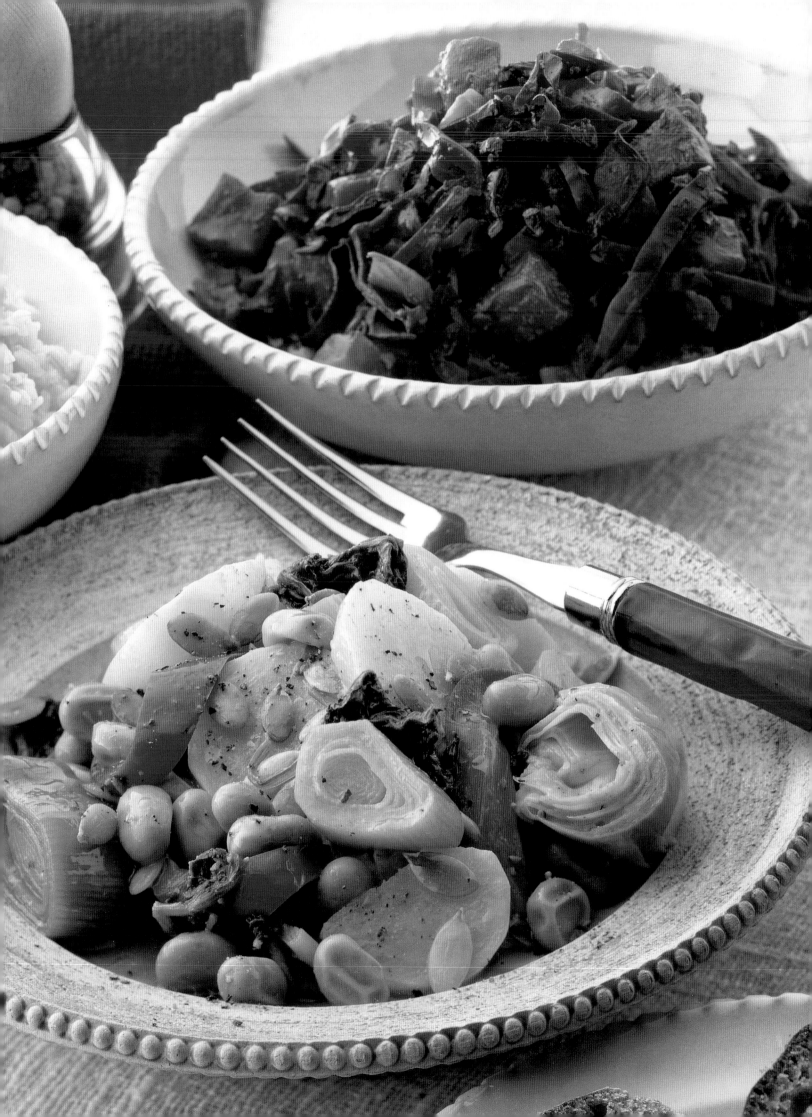

Purée of Lentils with Baked Eggs

This unusual dish makes an excellent vegetarian supper. If you prefer, bake the purée and eggs in one large baking dish.

INGREDIENTS

Serves 4

2 cups (1 pound) red lentils
3 leeks, thinly sliced
2 teaspoons coriander seeds, finely crushed
1 tablespoon chopped fresh cilantro
2 tablespoons chopped fresh mint
1 tablespoon red wine vinegar
4 cups vegetable broth
sea salt and ground black pepper
4 eggs
generous handful of fresh parsley, chopped, to garnish

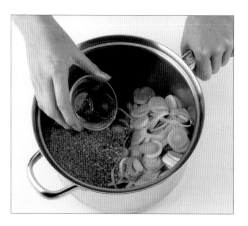

1 Put the lentils in a deep saucepan. Add the leeks, coriander seeds, fresh cilantro, mint, vinegar and broth. Bring to the boil, then lower the heat and simmer for 30–40 minutes, or until the lentils are cooked and have absorbed all the liquid.

2 Preheat the oven to 350°F. Season the lentils with salt and pepper and mix well. Spread out in 4 lightly greased individual baking dishes.

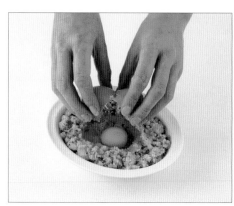

3 Using the back of a spoon, make a hollow in the lentil mixture in each dish. Break an egg into each hollow. Cover the dishes with foil and bake for 15–20 minutes, or until the eggs are set. Sprinkle with plenty of chopped parsley and serve at once.

NUTRITION NOTES

Per portion:

Calories	470
Fat, total	9.1g
saturated fat	2.2g
polyunsaturated fat	1.5g
monounsaturated fat	3.38g
Carbohydrate	65.8g
sugar, total	4.2g
starch	57.5g
Fiber – NSP	6.95g
Sodium	423.75mg

VARIATION

Spoon a 14-ounce can of chestnut purée into a bowl and beat it until softened. Stir the purée into the cooked lentil mixture, with extra broth if required. Proceed as in the main recipe.

Mushroom and Sunflower Seed Pie

Mushrooms, baby corn and spinach make a delectable filling for a pie, especially when sunflower seeds are included.

INGREDIENTS

Serves 6

1½ cups whole-wheat flour
6 tablespoons low-fat spread
3 tablespoons olive oil
6 ounces baby corn, each cut into 2–3 pieces
2 tablespoons sunflower seeds
2 cups (8 ounces) button mushrooms
3 ounces fresh spinach leaves, chopped
juice of 1 lemon
sea salt and ground black pepper
tomato salad, to serve

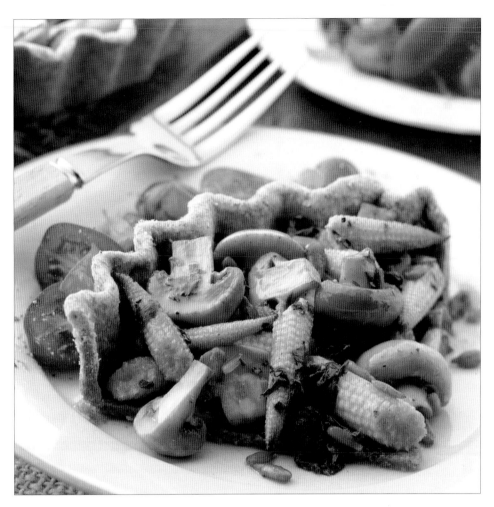

1 Preheat the oven to 350°F. Sift the flour into a bowl. Rub in the low-fat spread with your fingertips until the mixture resembles bread crumbs. Add just enough water to make a firm dough.

2 Roll out the dough on a lightly floured surface and use it to line a 9-inch pie pan. Prick the bottom with a fork, line the shell with foil and add a layer of beans or pastry weights. Bake for 15 minutes, then remove the foil and beans. Return the pastry shell to the oven and bake for another 10 minutes, or until crisp.

NUTRITION NOTES	
Per portion:	
Calories	250
Fat, total	16g
saturated fat	2.8g
polyunsaturated fat	3.85g
monounsaturated fat	8.25g
Carbohydrate	20.6g
sugar, total	1.45g
starch	19.1g
Fiber – NSP	4.05g
Sodium	434.5mg

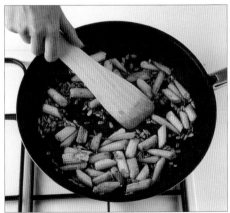

3 Meanwhile, heat the oil in a heavy frying pan. Fry the corn with the sunflower seeds for 5–8 minutes, until lightly browned all over.

COOK'S TIP

If the mushrooms are small, leave them whole or cut them in half or quarters.

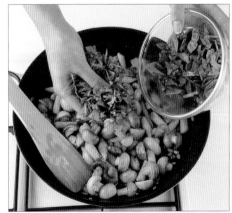

4 Add the button mushrooms, lower the heat slightly and cook the mixture for 2–3 minutes, then stir in the chopped spinach. Cover the pan and cook for 2–3 minutes.

5 Sharpen the filling with a little lemon juice. Add salt and pepper to taste. Spoon into the pastry shell. Serve warm or cold with a tomato salad.

Whole-Wheat Pasta with Caraway Cabbage

Crunchy cabbage and Brussels sprouts are the perfect partners for pasta in this healthy dish.

INGREDIENTS

Serves 6

6 tablespoons olive or sunflower oil
3 onions, roughly chopped
12 ounces green cabbage,
   roughly chopped
12 ounces Brussels sprouts, trimmed
   and halved
2 teaspoons caraway seeds
1 tablespoon chopped fresh dill
1²/₃ cups vegetable broth
sea salt and ground black pepper
1³/₄ cups (7 ounces) fresh or dried
   whole-wheat pasta spirals
dill sprigs, to garnish

1 Heat the oil in a large saucepan and fry the onions over low heat for 10 minutes, until softened.

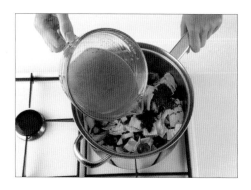

2 Add the cabbage and Brussels sprouts and cook for 2–3 minutes, then stir in the caraway seeds and chopped dill. Pour in the broth and season with salt and pepper to taste. Cover and simmer for 5–10 minutes, until the cabbage and sprouts are crisp-tender.

—— COOK'S TIP ——

If tiny baby Brussels sprouts are available, they can be used whole for this dish.

3 Meanwhile, cook the pasta in a pan of lightly salted boiling water until just tender.

4 Drain the pasta, put it into a bowl and add the cabbage mixture. Toss lightly, adjust the seasoning and serve garnished with dill sprigs.

—— NUTRITION NOTES ——	
Per portion:	
Calories	227
Fat, total	9.6g
saturated fat	1.4g
polyunsaturated fat	1.5g
monounsaturated fat	5.75g
Carbohydrate	30g
sugar, total	7.65g
starch	21.6g
Fiber – NSP	6.9g
Sodium	53.5mg

Cauliflower and Broccoli with Tomato Sauce

A low-fat alternative to cauliflower with cheese sauce. The addition of broccoli to the cauliflower gives extra color.

INGREDIENTS

Serves 6

1 onion, finely chopped
14-ounce can chopped tomatoes
3 tablespoons tomato paste
3 tablespoons whole-wheat flour
1¼ cups skim milk
1¼ cups water
sea salt and ground black pepper
6 cups mixed cauliflower and broccoli
   florets

1 Mix the onion, tomatoes and tomato paste in a small saucepan. Bring to a boil, lower the heat and simmer for 15–20 minutes.

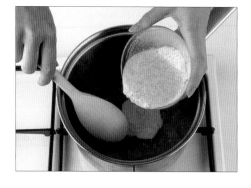

2 Mix the flour to a paste with a little of the milk. Stir the paste into the tomato mixture, then gradually add the remaining milk and the water. Stir constantly until the mixture boils and thickens. Season to taste with salt and pepper. Keep the sauce hot.

3 Steam the cauliflower and broccoli florets, covered, in a steamer over boiling water for 5–7 minutes, or until just tender. To serve, turn into a dish, pour the tomato sauce on top and sprinkle with extra pepper, if desired.

—— NUTRITION NOTES ——	
Per portion:	
Calories	116
Fat, total	1.85g
saturated fat	0.4g
polyunsaturated fat	0.9g
monounsaturated fat	0.2g
Carbohydrate	16.1g
sugar, total	10.3g
starch	5.4g
Fiber – NSP	4.5g
Sodium	86.8mg

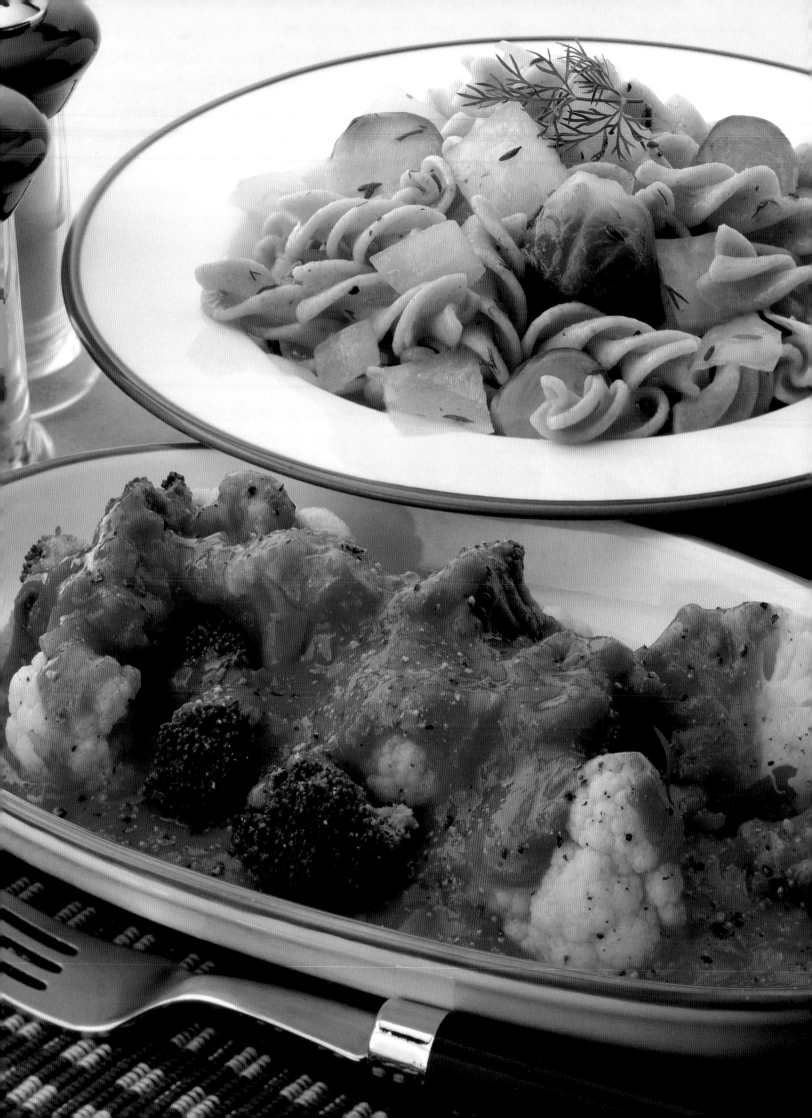

Red Pepper Risotto

The character of this delicious risotto depends on the type of rice you use. With Arborio rice, the risotto will be moist and creamy. If you use brown rice, reduce the amount of liquid for a drier dish with a nutty flavor.

INGREDIENTS

Serves 6
3 large red bell peppers
2 tablespoons olive oil
3 large garlic cloves, thinly sliced
14-ounce can chopped tomatoes
2 bay leaves
5–6¼ cups vegetable broth
2½ cups (1 pound) raw Arborio rice
    (Italian risotto rice) or brown rice
sea salt and ground black pepper
6 fresh basil leaves, chopped

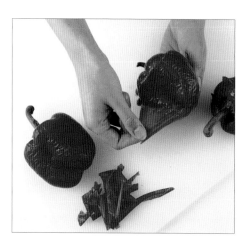

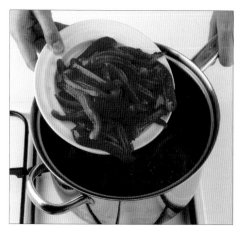

1 Preheat the broiler. Put the peppers in a broiler pan and broil until the skins are blistered all over, turning often. Put the peppers in a bowl, cover with several layers of damp paper towels and let sit for 10 minutes. Peel off the skins, then slice the peppers, discarding the cores and seeds.

2 Heat the oil in a large saucepan. Add the garlic and tomatoes and cook over gentle heat for 5 minutes, then add the pepper slices and bay leaves. Stir well and cook for 15 minutes more.

3 Pour the broth into another saucepan and heat it to a simmering point. Stir the rice into the vegetable mixture and cook for 2 minutes, then add two or three ladlefuls of the hot broth. Cook, stirring occasionally, until the broth has been absorbed.

4 Continue to add broth in this way, making sure each addition has been absorbed before pouring in the next. When the rice is tender, season with salt and pepper to taste. Remove the pan from the heat, cover and let stand for 10 minutes. Remove the bay leaves, then stir in the basil and serve.

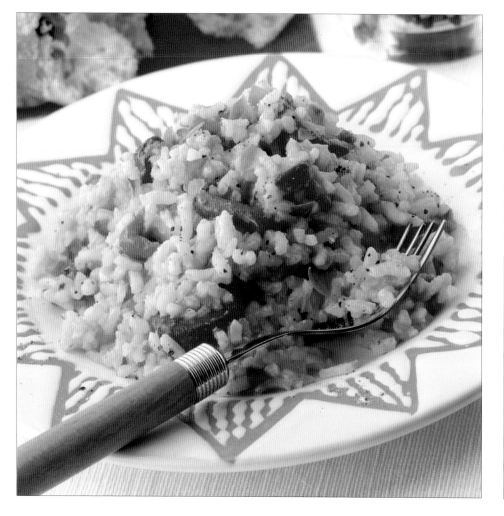

NUTRITION NOTES	
Per portion:	
Calories	387
Fat, total	10.75g
saturated fat	1.73g
polyunsaturated fat	1.3g
monounsaturated fat	6.3g
Carbohydrate	69.2g
sugar, total	7.85g
starch	60.85g
Fiber – NSP	3.2g
Sodium	645mg

Stir-fried Vegetables with Cashew Nuts

Stir-frying is the perfect way of making a delicious, colorful— and very speedy meal.

INGREDIENTS

Serves 4

2 pounds mixed vegetables
  (see Cook's Tip)
2–4 tablespoons sunflower or olive oil
2 garlic cloves, finely chopped
1 tablespoon grated fresh ginger
$\frac{1}{2}$ cup cashews or $\frac{1}{4}$ cup sunflower
  seeds, pumpkin seeds or sesame seeds
soy sauce
sea salt and ground black pepper

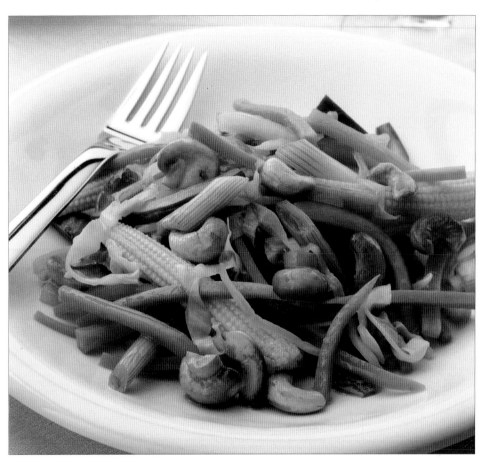

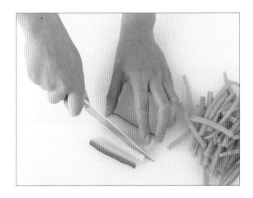

1 Cut the vegetables into uniform slices as required. Carrots and cucumber should be cut into matchsticks.

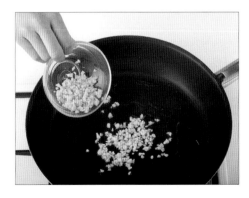

2 Heat a nonstick frying pan, then trickle the oil around the rim so that it runs down to coat the surface. When it is hot, add the garlic and ginger and cook for 2–3 minutes, stirring. Add the harder vegetables and stir-fry for 5 minutes, until they start to soften.

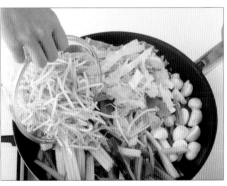

3 Add the softer vegetables and stir-fry over medium-high heat for about 3–4 minutes until just crisp-tender.

COOK'S TIP

Use a pack of stir-fry vegetables or make up your own mixture. Choose from carrots, snow peas, baby corn, bok choy, cucumber, bean sprouts, mushrooms, bell peppers and scallions. Drained canned bamboo shoots and water chestnuts are delicious additions.

4 Stir in the cashews or seeds. Season with soy sauce, salt and pepper to taste. Serve at once.

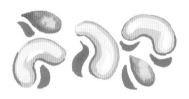

NUTRITION NOTES

Per portion:

Calories	288
Fat, total	21.3g
saturated fat	2.4g
polyunsaturated fat	8.3g
monounsaturated fat	9.3g
Carbohydrate	15.8g
sugar, total	9g
starch	5.2g
Fiber – NSP	5g
Sodium	170mg

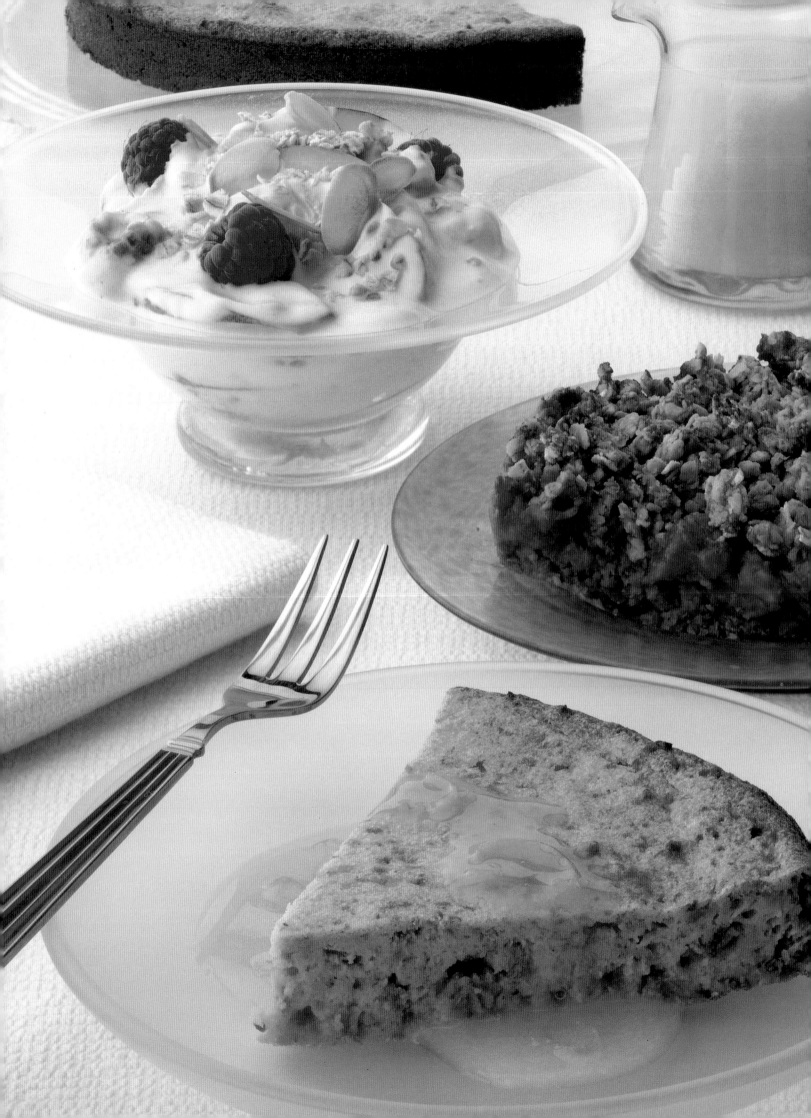

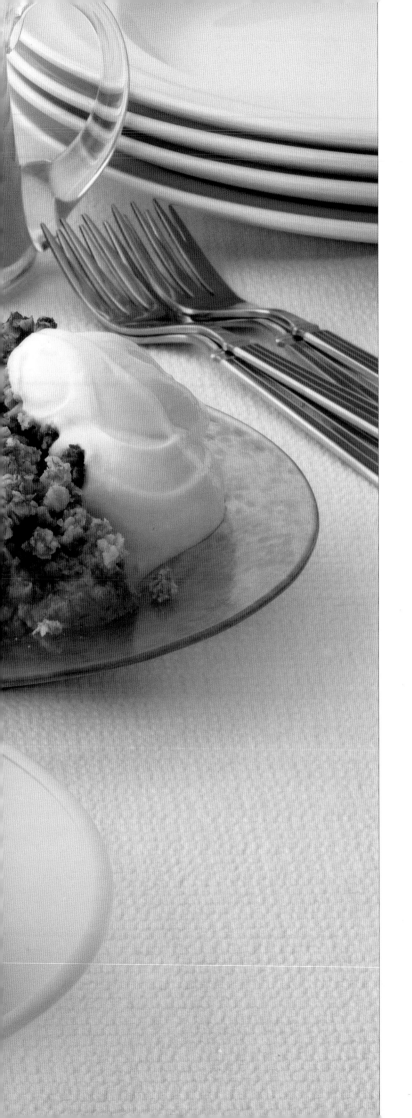

DESSERTS

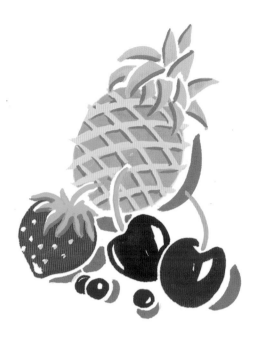

Desserts are always thought to be a no-go area for diabetics, but modern advice and the judicious use of fruits mean that diabetics can now eat a wonderful range of desserts. Try, for example, a fruit tart with a tasty yogurt topping, a crumbly oat layer with a strawberry filling or a delectable orange cheesecake. The recipes here are sweetened with fruits rather than sugar alternatives, which means that diabetics can absorb the sugar more easily. Nonetheless, it is important to remember that most desserts should be eaten only as occasional treats.

Baked Fruit Tart

Crisp pastry, juicy baked fruit and a delectable creamy yogurt and almond topping make this tart a family favorite.

INGREDIENTS

Serves 6
1 cup whole-wheat flour
$^1/_2$ cup gram flour or besan
4 tablespoons low-fat spread
about 3 tablespoons cold water

For the filling and topping
1 tablespoon liquid pear and
    apple concentrate
1 cooking apple
2 large oranges
3 kiwifruit
1$^1/_4$ cups low-fat plain yogurt
1 tablespoon sliced almonds, toasted

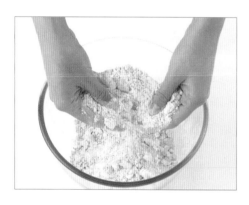

1 Preheat the oven to 350°F. Mix the whole-wheat and gram flours in a large mixing bowl and rub in the low-fat spread with your fingertips until the mixture resembles coarse bread crumbs. Add just enough of the cold water to make a soft dough.

COOK'S TIP

To toast the almonds, spread them out in a broiler pan and place them several inches away from the heat. Cook them until they are golden brown, stirring once or twice to make sure they brown on all sides. The process takes only a few minutes at most, so watch them closely in case they char.

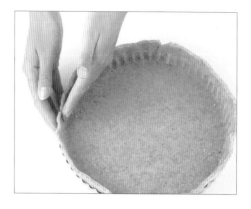

2 Roll out the pastry on a lightly floured surface and use it to line an 8-inch round tart pan.

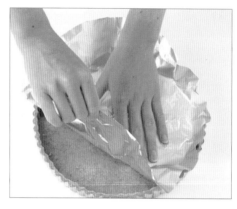

3 Prick the base of the pastry shell with a fork, line it with foil and add a layer of beans or pie weights. Bake for 15 minutes, then remove the foil and beans. Bake for 10 minutes more, until crisp. Remove the pastry shell from the oven, but leave the oven on.

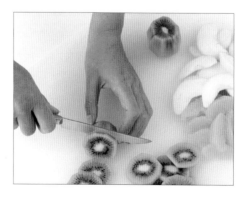

4 Carefully spread the pear and apple concentrate on the bottom of the pastry shell. Peel and slice the apple, oranges and kiwifruit.

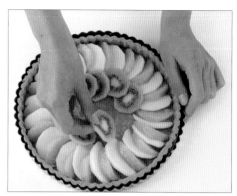

5 Arrange the fruit in the pastry shell, cover with foil and then bake for 20 minutes more. Let cool slightly.

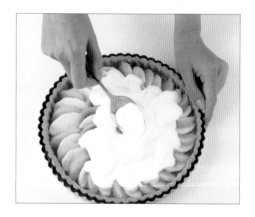

6 Spoon the yogurt over the fruit in an even layer. Sprinkle the sliced almonds over the top. Serve the tart warm or at room temperature.

NUTRITION NOTES

Per portion:

Calories	254
Fat, total	10.5g
saturated fat	3.8g
polyunsaturated fat	1.9g
monounsaturated fat	3.8g
Carbohydrate	31.9g
sugar, total	12.4g
starch	19.3g
Fiber – NSP	5g
Sodium	98mg

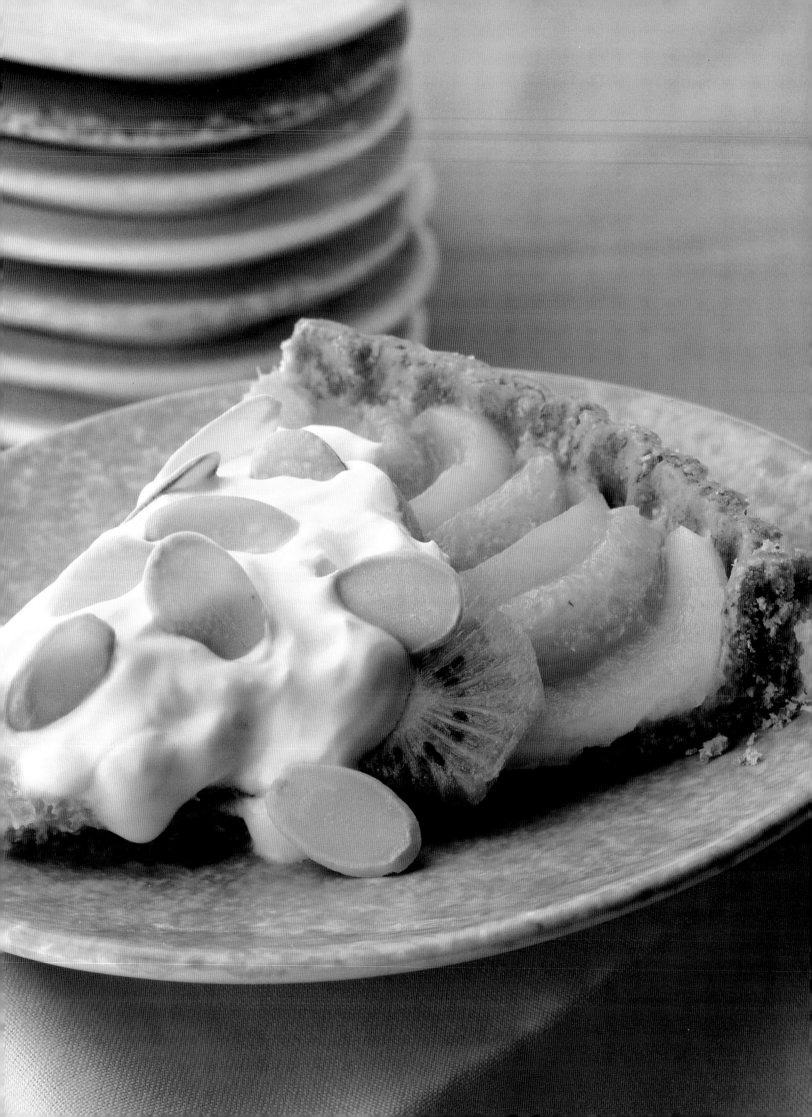

Hot Fruit Compote

The sugar content of this dessert is quite high, so serve it in small quantities along with a generous dollop of plain yogurt.

Ingredients

Serves 8

2½ cups (1 pound) mixed dried fruit, such as apricots, apples, prunes, raisins, golden raisins, figs and pears
2 cups water, plus additional
thinly slivered rind of 1 small lemon or 2 tablespoons lemon juice
1 cinnamon stick
low-fat plain yogurt, to serve

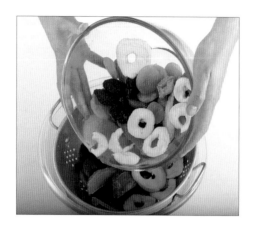

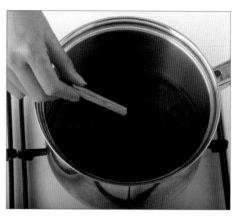

1 Soak the fruit in the 2 cups water about 8 hours or overnight, then drain, reserving the liquid.

2 Add additional water to the reserved liquid to make 2 cups. Add the lemon rind or juice and the cinnamon.

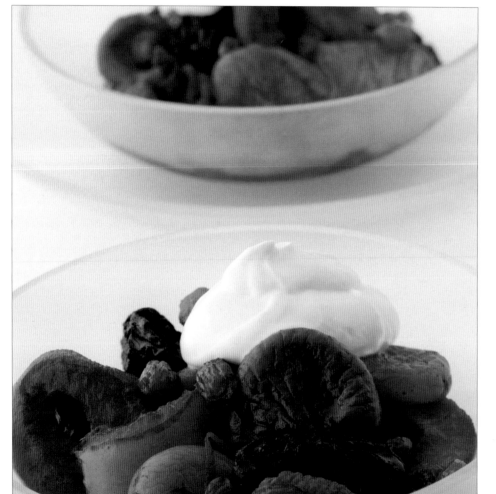

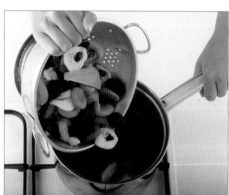

3 Bring to a boil, lower the heat and add the drained fruit. Simmer for 15 minutes, until the fruit is tender. Using a slotted spoon, transfer the fruit to a bowl. Simmer the syrup in the pan for 20 minutes, until reduced slightly and thickened. Pour it over the fruit. Serve warm, with yogurt.

Nutrition Notes	
Per portion:	
Calories	118
Fat, total	0.35g
saturated fat	0g
polyunsaturated fat	0.05g
monounsaturated fat	0g
Carbohydrate	28.9g
sugar, total	28.9g
starch	0g
Fiber – NSP	4.6g
Sodium	15.1mg

Italian Fruit Salad and Ice Cream

If you visit Italy in the summer you will find little sidewalk fruit stands selling small dishes of macerated soft fruits, which are delectable on their own, but also make a wonderful ice cream.

INGREDIENTS

Serves 6

8 cups (2 pounds) mixed soft fruits, such as strawberries, raspberries, blueberries, peaches, apricots, plums and melon
juice of 3–4 oranges
juice of 1 lemon
1 tablespoon liquid pear and apple concentrate
4 tablespoons whipping cream
2 tablespoons orange-flavored liqueur (optional)
mint sprigs, to garnish

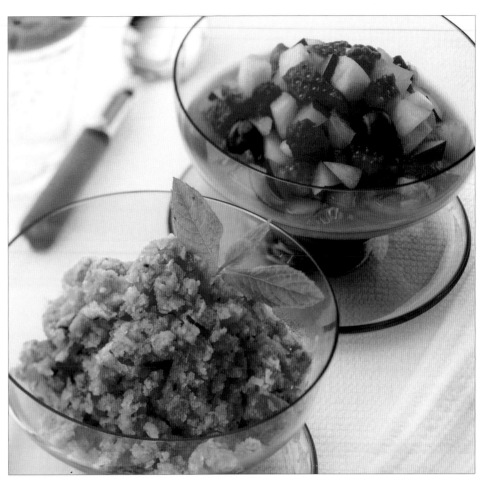

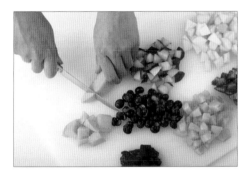

1 Prepare the fruit. Leave small berries whole; cut larger fruit into reasonably small pieces, but not so small that the mixture becomes a mush.

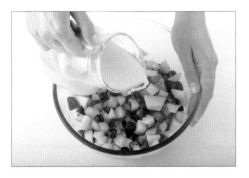

2 Put the fruit pieces in a serving bowl and add enough orange juice to cover. Add the lemon juice, stir gently, cover and chill for 2 hours.

3 Set half the macerated fruit aside to serve as it is. Purée the remainder in a blender or food processor.

--- COOK'S TIP ---

The macerated fruit makes a delicious drink. Purée, then press through a strainer.

--- NUTRITION NOTES ---

Per portion:

Calories	105
Fat, total	4.1g
saturated fat	2.5g
polyunsaturated fat	0.15g
monounsaturated fat	1.15g
Carbohydrate	13.5g
sugar, total	13.5g
starch	0g
Fiber – NSP	2.95g
Sodium	12.85mg

4 Gently warm the pear and apple concentrate and stir it into the fruit purée. Whip the cream and fold it in, then add the liqueur, if using.

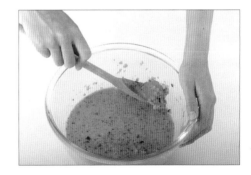

5 Churn the mixture in an ice-cream maker. Alternatively, place it in a suitable container for freezing. Freeze until ice crystals form around the edge, then beat the mixture until smooth. Repeat the process once or twice, then freeze until firm. Soften slightly before serving in scoops garnished with mint, accompanied by the macerated fruit.

Cranberry Rice Pudding

INGREDIENTS

Serves 4

1¼ cups unsweetened rice milk
1 vanilla bean
¼ cup (2 ounces) raw short-grain rice
¼ cup cranberries

— NUTRITION NOTES —	
Per portion:	
Calories	71
Fat, total	1.6g
saturated fat	0.3g
polyunsaturated fat	0.8g
monounsaturated fat	0.4g
Carbohydrate	12g
sugar, total	1g
starch	11g
Fiber – NSP	0.4g
Sodium	25mg

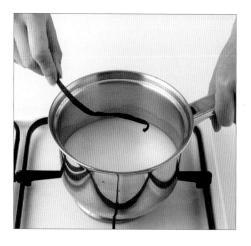

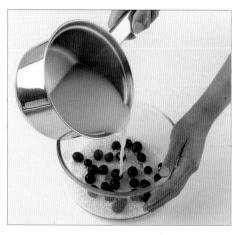

1 Preheat the oven to 300°F. Pour the rice milk into a small saucepan and add the vanilla bean. Bring the milk to just below boiling point, then remove the saucepan from the heat and let the milk and vanilla infuse for 10 minutes.

2 Put the rice and cranberries in a baking dish. Remove the vanilla bean from the milk, pour the milk into the dish and stir gently to mix lightly. Bake for 2½–3 hours, stirring from time to time. Serve the pudding warm or let sit until cool.

Banana and Pineapple Ice Cream

INGREDIENTS

Serves 4

1 banana
5 ounces fresh pineapple chunks
⅔ cup low-fat plain yogurt
⅔ cup whipping cream, lightly
  whipped
mint sprigs, to garnish

— NUTRITION NOTES —	
Per portion:	
Calories	200
Fat, total	15.2g
saturated fat	9.5g
polyunsaturated fat	0.5g
monounsaturated fat	4.5g
Carbohydrate	13.5g
sugar, total	13g
starch	0.6g
Fiber – NSP	0.7g
Sodium	47mg

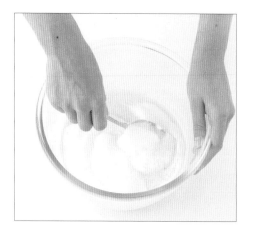

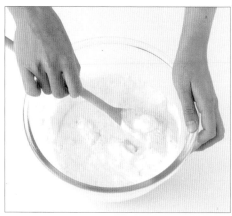

1 Purée the banana and pineapple in a blender or food processor. Pour the purée into a large bowl and stir in the plain yogurt. Fold in the cream.

2 Churn the mixture in an ice-cream maker. Alternatively, place it in a suitable container for freezing. Freeze until ice crystals form around the edges. Process or beat the mixture until it is smooth, then return it to the freezer.

3 Repeat the process once or twice, then freeze until firm. Remove from the freezer to soften slightly before serving, garnished with mint.

— VARIATION —

Substitute the same quantity of drained canned pineapple in fruit juice for the fresh pineapple, or use fresh mango instead.

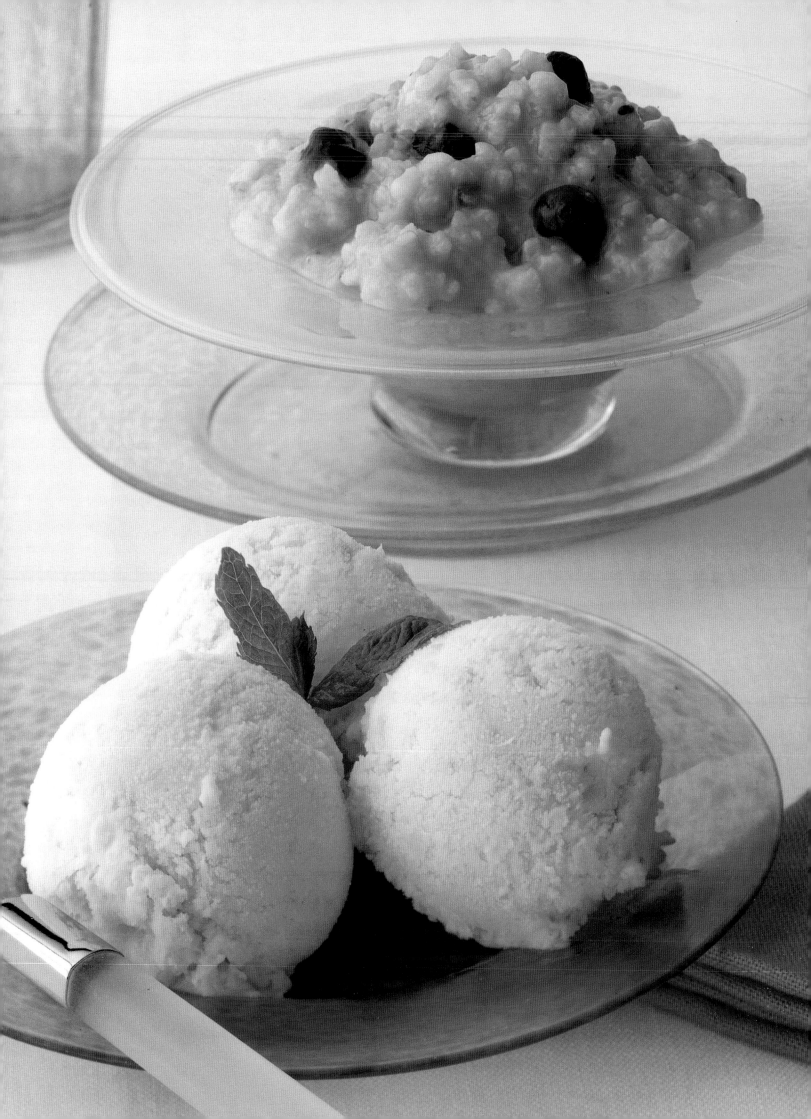

Apple and Banana Crumble

An old favorite, this crumble is naturally sweet, with a crisp topping contrasting beautifully with the soft fruit. Bananas are delicious in a crumble and served with low-fat yogurt.

INGREDIENTS

Serves 6

2 large cooking apples
2 large bananas
4 tablespoons water
4 tablespoons (¼ cup) low-fat spread
2–3 tablespoons pear and apple spread
¼ cup whole-wheat flour
1 cup rolled oats
2 tablespoons sunflower seeds
low-fat yogurt, to serve (optional)

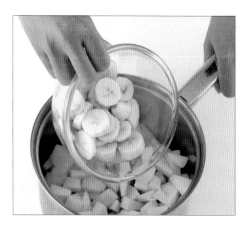

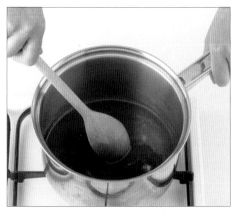

1 Preheat the oven to 350°F. Cut the apples into quarters, remove the cores, then chop the apples into small pieces, leaving the skin on. Peel and slice the bananas. Mix the apples, bananas and water in a saucepan and cook until soft and pulpy.

2 Melt the low-fat spread with the pear and apple spread in a separate pan. Off the heat, stir in the flour, oats and sunflower seeds and mix well.

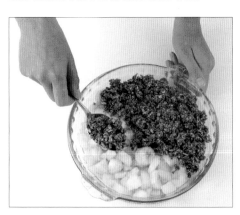

3 Transfer the apple and banana mixture to an 8-inch baking dish and spread the oat crumble over the top. Bake for about 20 minutes, or until the topping is golden brown. Serve warm or at room temperature, alone or with low-fat yogurt.

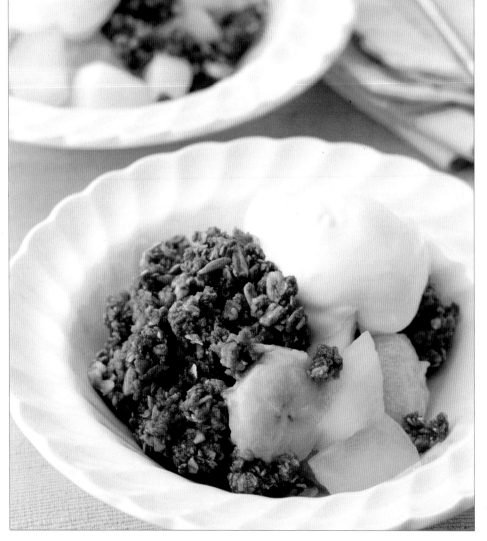

NUTRITION NOTES	
Per portion:	
Calories	181
Fat, total	7.36g
saturated fat	1.5g
polyunsaturated fat	2.9g
monounsaturated fat	2.5g
Carbohydrate	28.5g
sugar, total	12g
starch	16.3g
Fiber – NSP	3.2g
Sodium	58mg

Chocolate and Orange Mousse

There's no hint of deprivation in this divine dessert! It makes a great occasional treat, but eat it with a high-fiber main course.

INGREDIENTS

Serves 8

6 ounces good-quality bittersweet
  chocolate, broken into squares
grated rind and juice of 1½ large
  oranges, plus extra slivered rind
  for garnish
1 teaspoon unflavored gelatin
4 eggs, separated
6 tablespoons unsweetened soy cream
4 tablespoons brandy
chopped pistachio nuts, to garnish

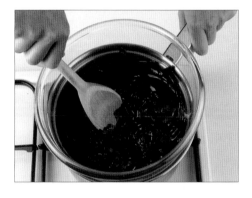

1 Melt the chocolate in a heatproof bowl over a pan of simmering water. Put 2 tablespoons of the orange juice in a heatproof bowl and sprinkle the gelatin on top. When the gelatin is softened, set the bowl over a pan of hot water and stir until it has dissolved.

NUTRITION NOTES	
Per portion:	
Calories	230
Fat, total	12.4g
saturated fat	4.6g
polyunsaturated fat	0.6g
monounsaturated fat	3.4g
Carbohydrate	17.3g
sugar, total	17g
Starch	0.2g
Fiber – NSP	0.55g
Sodium	113mg

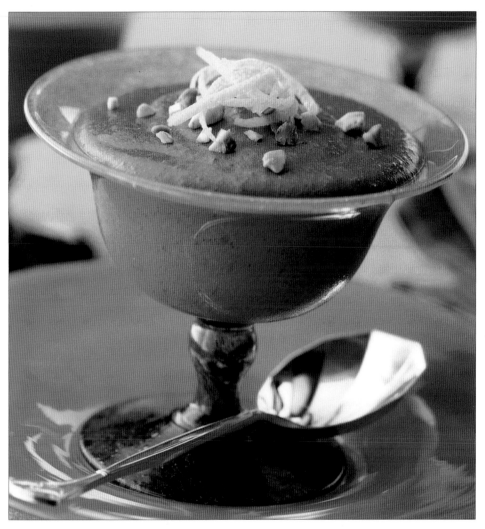

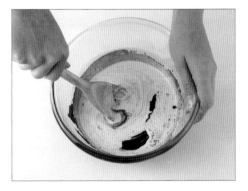

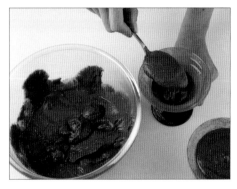

2 Let the chocolate cool slightly, then beat in the orange rind, egg yolks, soy cream and brandy, followed by the gelatin mixture and the remaining orange juice. Set aside.

3 Beat the egg whites in a grease-free bowl until they form soft peaks, then gently fold them into the chocolate and orange mixture.

4 Spoon or pour the mixture into six sundae dishes or glasses, or into a single glass bowl. Cover and chill until the mousse sets. Garnish with the chopped pistachio nuts and extra slivered orange rind before serving.

Steamed Orange and Lemon Pudding

This delicious old-fashioned pudding tastes so good that you won't begrudge the time spent steaming it.

INGREDIENTS

Serves 8
²/₃ cup raisins
4 tablespoons brandy
²/₃ cup pitted dates
8 tablespoons (½ cup) low-fat spread
2 oranges
2 lemons
2 cups whole-wheat flour
1 tablespoon baking powder
3 eggs
1 pear, about 4 ounces, peeled, cored and puréed
1 cup low-fat fromage frais

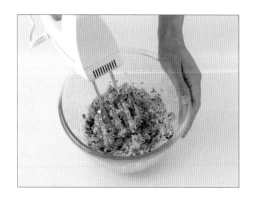

1 Soak the raisins in the brandy in a small bowl. Meanwhile, put the dates in a separate bowl, add enough boiling water to cover them and let soak for 10 minutes. Drain the dates, chop them finely and place in a mixing bowl. Add the low-fat spread. Grate the rind from the oranges and lemons and add it to the bowl. Beat well.

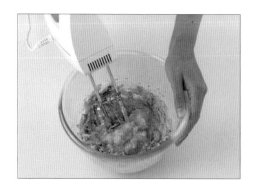

2 Sift the flour with the baking powder. Gradually beat the eggs and pear purée into the creamed mixture, adding a little of the flour mixture if the mixture looks curdled.

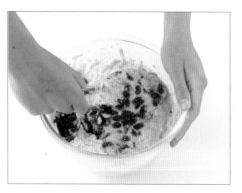

3 Fold in the rest of the flour mixture, then the raisins, along with any remaining brandy. Spoon the mixture into a greased 1-quart pudding bowl. It should be about two-thirds full.

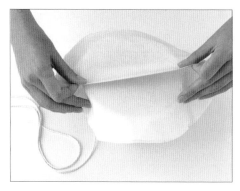

4 Cover the pudding bowl with a pleated double layer of waxed paper tied firmly in place with string.

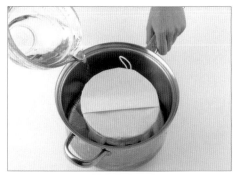

5 Set the pudding bowl on an inverted saucer in a large saucepan. Pour in enough boiling water to come halfway up the sides of the bowl. Cover the saucepan tightly.

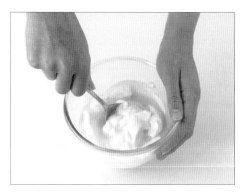

6 Steam the pudding in gently simmering water for 1½–2 hours, topping up the water from time to time. Squeeze the juice from one of the oranges and both the lemons. Put the fromage frais in a bowl and gradually beat in the citrus juice. Turn the pudding out onto a warmed serving plate and serve with the citrus sauce.

NUTRITION NOTES	
Per portion:	
Calories	303
Fat, total	8.8g
saturated fat	2.4g
polyunsaturated fat	1.85g
monounsaturated fat	3.65g
Carbohydrate	45g
sugar, total	23.9g
starch	21.15g
Fibre – NSP	2.4g
Sodium	323mg

Peach and Raspberry Yogurt Fool

Low-fat, low-sugar plain or fruit yogurt makes an excellent basis for this delicious, quick and healthy dessert.

INGREDIENTS

Serves 4
2 peaches
8 ounces raspberries
2½ cups low-fat plain or low-fat, low-sugar fruit yogurt
4 teaspoons rolled oats
4 teaspoons sliced almonds

1 Cut the peaches in half, remove the pits and then slice the flesh into thin wedges.

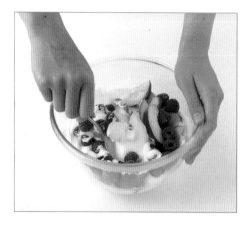

2 Mix the peaches and raspberries with the yogurt in a bowl, then spoon into 4 sundae glasses and chill.

3 Spread out the rolled oats and almonds in a broiler pan. Broil them until lightly toasted, shaking the pan frequently. Cool, then sprinkle the oat mixture over the dessert and serve.

VARIATION

This works well with strawberries, apricots, kiwifruit, pears, bananas or pineapple chunks. Match with a fruit yogurt of the same flavor, or a complementary variety.

NUTRITION NOTES

Per portion:

Calories	165
Fat, total	4.65g
saturated fat	1.1g
polyunsaturated fat	0.95g
monounsaturated fat	2.25g
Carbohydrate	21.65g
sugar, total	18.3g
starch	3.4g
Fiber – NSP	2.95g
Sodium	128mg

Strawberry Oat Crunch

This looks good and tastes delicious. The strawberries form a tasty filling between the layers of oat crumble.

INGREDIENTS

Serves 6
1¼ cups rolled oats
½ cup whole-wheat flour
6 tablespoons low-fat spread
2 tablespoons liquid pear and apple concentrate
1¼ pounds strawberries
2 teaspoons arrowroot
low-fat plain yogurt or unsweetened soy cream, to serve

VARIATION

Use dried apricots (chop half and cook the rest to a purée with a little apple juice). Add chopped almonds to the crumble.

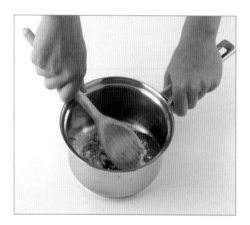

1 Preheat the oven to 350°F. Mix the oats and flour in a bowl. Melt the low-fat spread with the concentrate in a saucepan; stir into the bowl.

2 Purée half the berries in a food processor; chop the rest. Mix the arrowroot with a little of the purée in a small saucepan, then add the rest of the purée. Heat gently until thickened, stirring, then stir in the chopped berries.

3 Spread half the oat crumble mixture over the bottom of a 7-inch round shallow baking dish to form a layer at least ½ inch thick. Top with the strawberry mixture, then the remaining crumble, patting it down gently. Bake the crunch for 30 minutes. Serve warm or cold, alone or with low-fat yogurt or soy cream.

NUTRITION NOTES

Per portion:

Calories	208
Fat, total	7.65g
saturated fat	1.85g
polyunsaturated fat	2.25g
monounsaturated fat	3.05g
Carbohydrate	31.35g
sugar, total	8.4g
starch	22.95g
Fiber – NSP	3.45g
Sodium	89.35

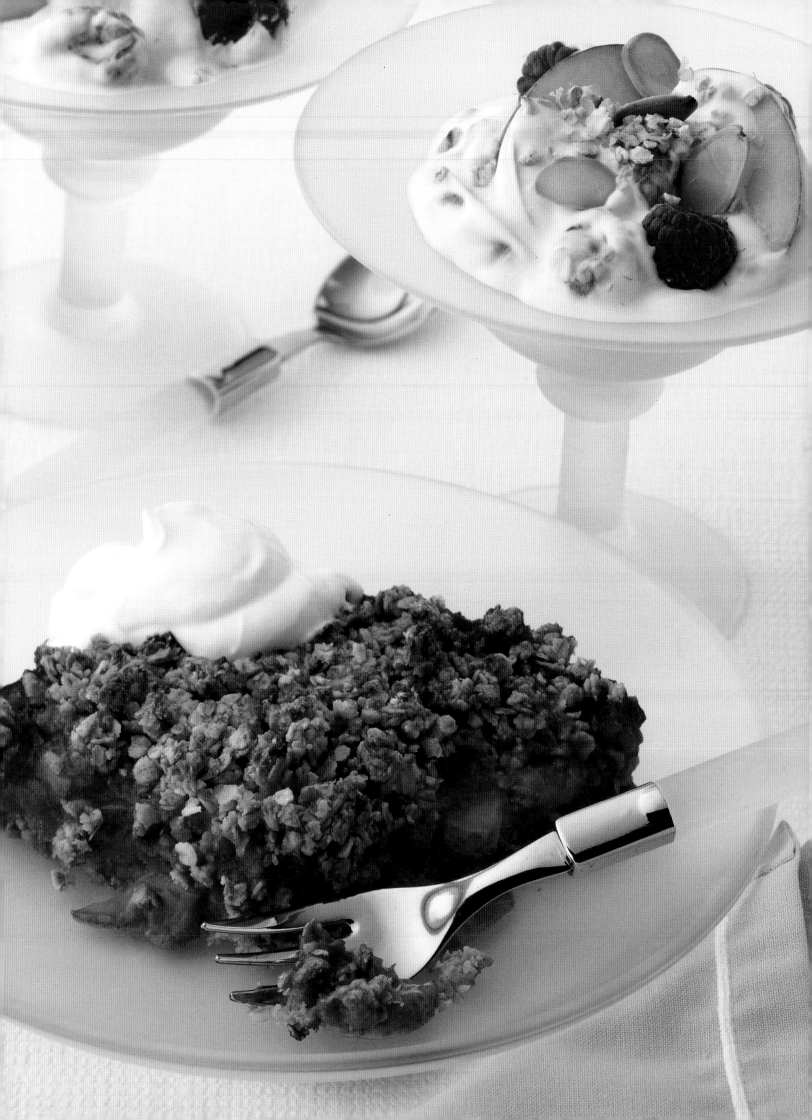

Plum, Apple and Banana Biscuit Pie

This is one of those simple, satisfying desserts that everyone enjoys. It is delicious hot or cold, served on its own or with yogurt.

INGREDIENTS

Serves 4

1 pound plums
1 tart cooking apple, about 4 ounces
1 large banana
²/₃ cup water
1 cup whole-wheat flour, or half whole-wheat and half all-purpose flour
2 teaspoons baking powder
3 tablespoons raisins
4 tablespoons buttermilk or low-fat plain yogurt
low-fat plain yogurt, to serve

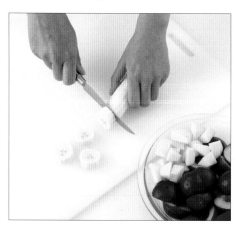

1 Preheat the oven to 350°F. Cut the plums in half and ease out the pits. Peel, core and chop the apple, then peel and slice the banana.

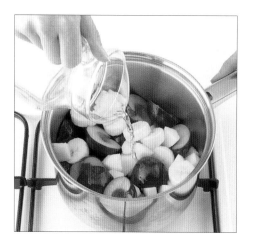

2 Mix the plums, apple and banana in a saucepan. Pour in the water. Bring to a simmer and cook gently for 15 minutes, or until the fruit is soft.

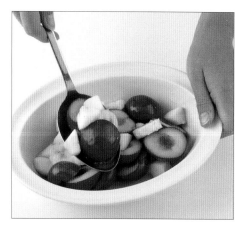

3 Spoon the fruit mixture into a baking dish. Level the surface.

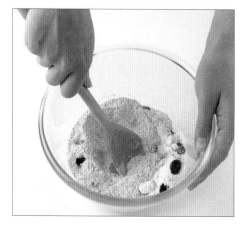

4 Mix the flour, baking powder and raisins in a bowl. Add the buttermilk or yogurt and mix to a very soft dough.

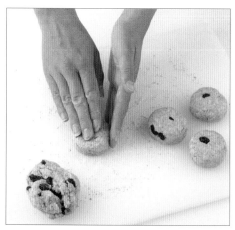

5 Transfer the biscuit dough to a lightly floured surface and divide it into 6–8 portions, then pat each into a flattish biscuit.

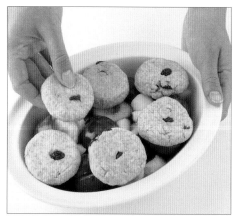

6 Cover the plum and apple mixture with the biscuits. Bake the pie for 40 minutes, until the biscuits are cooked through. Serve the pie hot with plain yogurt, or let it sit until cool.

NUTRITION NOTES	
Per portion:	
Calories	195
Fat, total	1g
saturated fat	0.2g
polyunsaturated fat	0.35g
monounsaturated fat	0.1g
Carbohydrate	43.6g
sugar, total	24.2g
starch	19.4g
Fiber – NSP	5.2g
Sodium	315.2mg

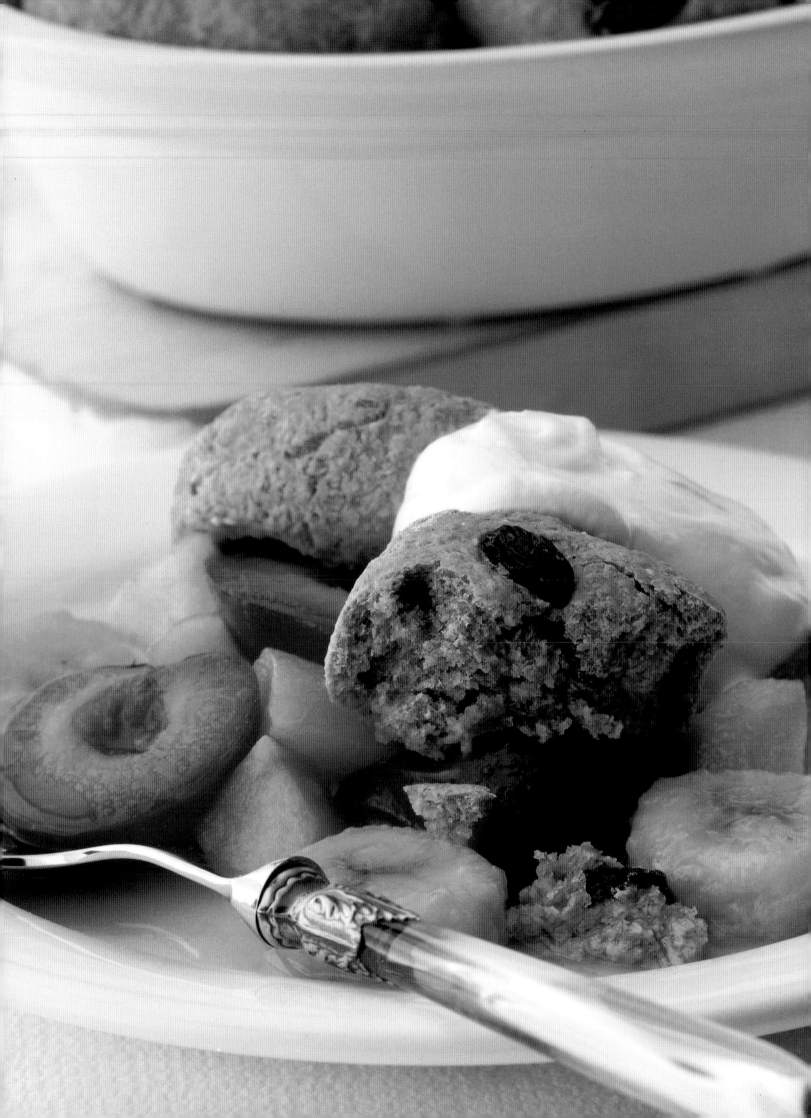

Baked Orange Cheesecake

Making this delicious baked cheesecake couldn't be simpler; there's no crumb crust. The flavorful orange-cheese filling is matched with a tangy sauce.

INGREDIENTS

Serves 8
4 oranges
1 cup low-fat fromage frais
²⁄₃ cup ground almonds
¹⁄₃ cup potato flour
2 teaspoons almond extract
¹⁄₂ teaspoon grated nutmeg
3 eggs, separated
²⁄₃ cup golden raisins
1 teaspoon arrowroot

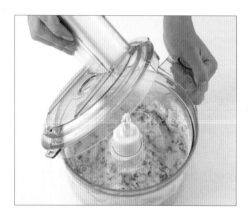

1 Preheat the oven to 350°F. Grate the rind from one orange and squeeze the orange. Place the rind and juice in a food processor with the fromage frais, ground almonds, potato flour, almond extract and nutmeg. Process briefly, then transfer to a large mixing bowl.

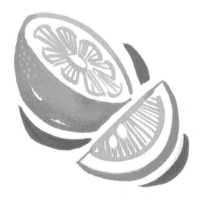

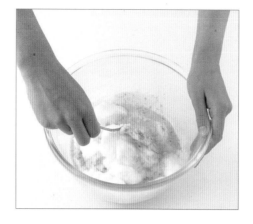

2 Beat in the egg yolks and golden raisins. Beat the egg whites in a clean grease-free bowl, then fold them into the creamy mixture.

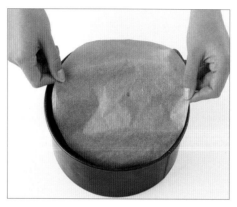

3 Line an 8-inch springform cake pan with baking parchment or waxed paper. Grease the paper lightly, then pour in the batter. Bake for 40 minutes, until the cheesecake has risen and set.

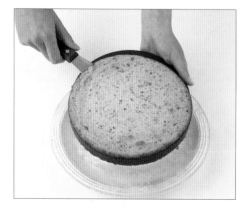

4 Set the cheesecake aside in the pan on a wire rack to cool, then unclip and remove the sides of the pan. Carefully slide the dessert onto a serving dish.

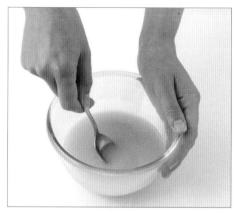

5 Put the arrowroot in a small bowl. Grate the rind from two of the remaining oranges, then squeeze all the remaining fruit. Add a little juice to the arrowroot to make a paste, then stir in the rest of the juice and the rind.

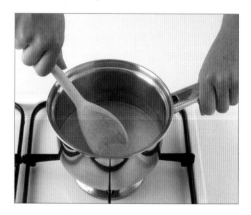

6 Pour the mixture into a saucepan and heat gently, stirring all the time, until the mixture thickens slightly. Cool the sauce to room temperature, then serve it with the cheesecake.

NUTRITION NOTES

Per portion:

Calories	181
Fat, total	6.3g
saturated fat	1.15g
polyunsaturated fat	1.2g
monounsaturated fat	3.3g
Carbohydrate	24.6g
sugar, total	19.35g
starch	5.35g
Fiber – NSP	2.45g
Sodium	51mg

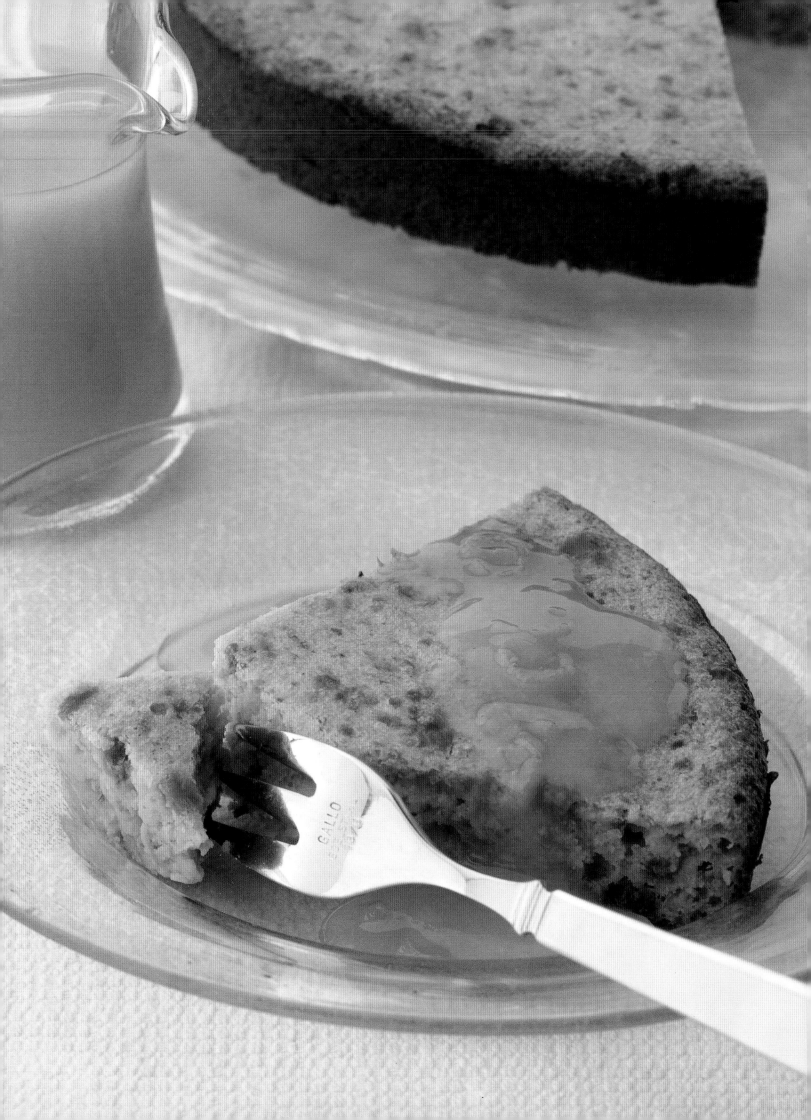

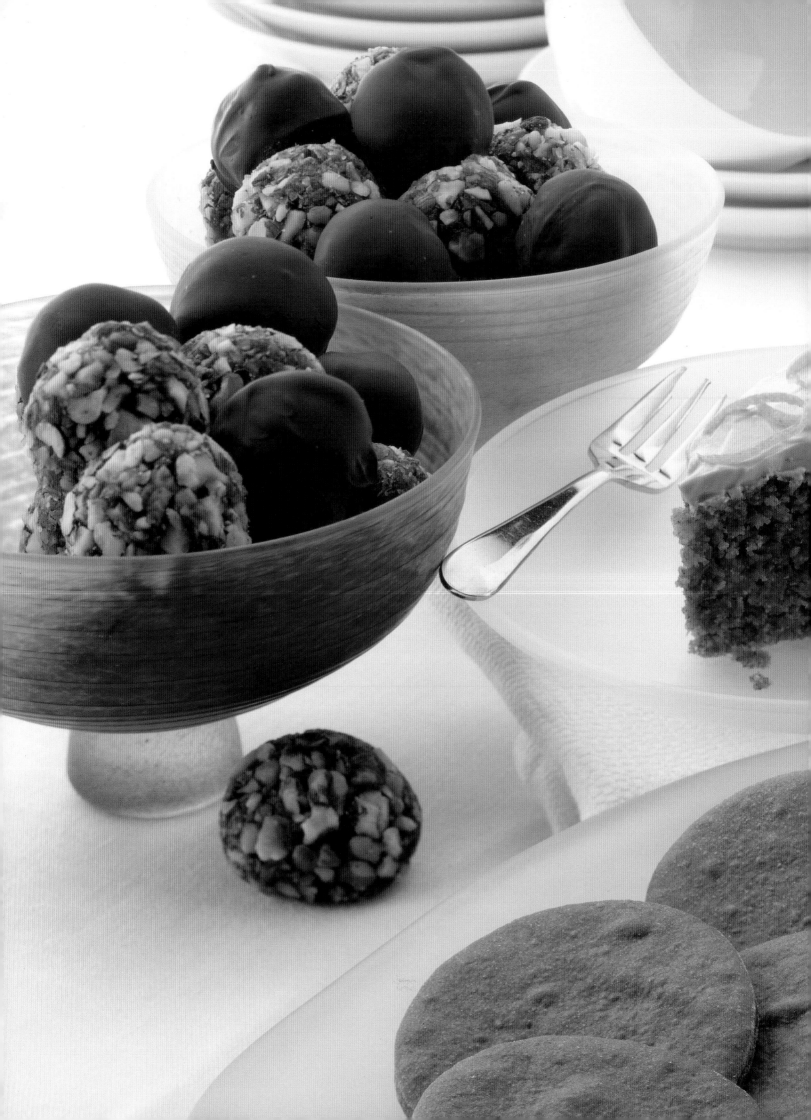

CAKES, BAKED GOODS AND CANDIES

Fancy morning-coffee biscuits, afternoon cakes and even after-dinner sweets are no longer off the menu for diabetics, although they still need to be included in a daily allocation of carbohydrates. Pine Nut Cookies and Ginger Cookies make good snacks for children as well as delicious coffee accompaniments. Cakes flavored with apple and spices or chocolate and prunes use fruits instead of sugar, as do the Fruit and Nut Chocolates and Apple and Date Balls. (Note: Where recipes have a nutritional breakdown for the whole cake, divide them into whatever size portions you want and calculate accordingly.)

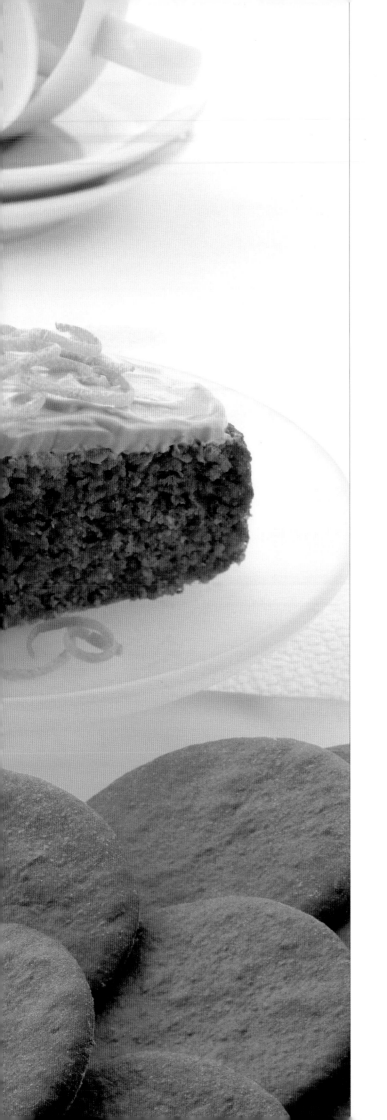

Passion Cake

Grated carrot keeps this cake beautifully moist while adding to the sweetness of the fruit.

INGREDIENTS

Makes an 8-inch cake
8 tablespoons (½ cup) low-fat spread
3 eggs, beaten
⅔ cup pitted dates, softened in boiling water if necessary
1 large carrot, about 5 ounces, finely grated
1 large pear, about 6 ounces, peeled, cored and puréed
1½ cups whole-wheat flour
2 teaspoons baking powder
2 teaspoons ground cinnamon
1 teaspoon grated nutmeg
½ teaspoon ground allspice
½ teaspoon salt
slivered orange rind, to decorate

For the icing
2 tablespoons pear and apple spread
scant 1 cup low-fat fromage frais
grated rind of 1 orange

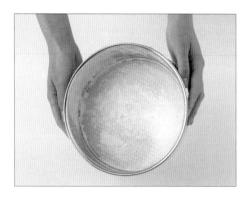

1 Preheat the oven to 375°F. Lightly grease and flour an 8-inch springform cake pan.

COOK'S TIP

A food processor makes short work of preparing the carrot and pear. Use the finest grater attachment for the carrot, then switch to the stainless steel blade and purée the chopped (uncooked) pear flesh.

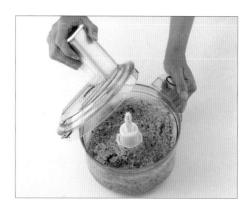

2 Cream the low-fat spread in a bowl. Gradually beat in the eggs and dates. Mix in the grated carrot and the pear purée. Alternatively, use a food processor to mix the ingredients, then transfer to a bowl.

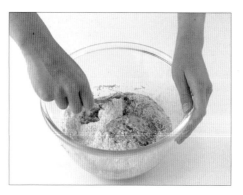

3 Sift the flour with the baking powder, spices and salt, then fold the dry ingredients gently but thoroughly into the creamed mixture.

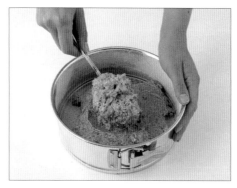

4 Spoon the batter into the prepared springform pan. Bake for 25 minutes, or until the cake is firm to the touch. Remove the sides of the pan and transfer the cake to a wire rack. Allow it to cool completely before icing it.

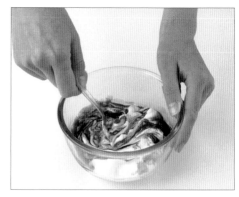

5 To make the icing for the cake, heat the pear and apple spread in a small saucepan until it is just runny. Put the fromage frais in a bowl. Stir in the melted pear and apple spread and the grated orange rind.

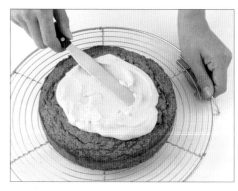

6 Spread the icing evenly over the cake. Decorate the top with the slivered orange rind and allow to set.

NUTRITION NOTES

Per cake:

Calories	1,520
Fat, total	73g
saturated fat	20g
polyunsaturated fat	16g
monounsaturated fat	30g
Carbohydrate	176g
sugar, total	63g
starch	112g
Fiber – NSP	24.8g
Sodium	2,264mg

Lemon and Walnut Cake

Don't stint on the lemon rind—it gives this cake a wonderful zesty tang that complements the flavor of the walnuts.

INGREDIENTS

Makes an 8-inch cake
1 large banana, about 5 ounces
16 tablespoonss (1 cup) low-fat spread
scant 1 cup pitted dates
5 eggs
2 3/4 cups whole-wheat flour,
   or half whole-wheat and half
   all-purpose flour
3/4 cup walnut pieces
4 large lemons

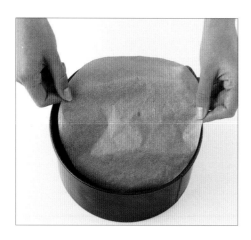

1 Preheat the oven to 350°F. Lightly grease a deep 8-inch removable-bottomed or springform cake pan. Line the bottom of the pan with baking parchment or waxed paper.

COOK'S TIPS

If the dates are very hard, soften them in a bowl of boiling water for 10 minutes before draining and using.

Make sure that you buy plain dates for cooking and eating, not the kind that are chopped and coated with sugar.

Look for packages of walnut pieces in supermarkets, as they are usually much less expensive than either shelled walnuts or walnut halves.

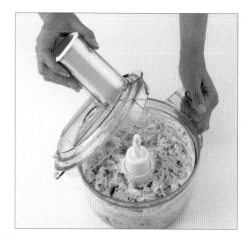

2 Peel and chop the banana. Process with the low-fat spread and dates.

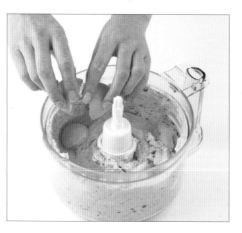

3 Add 1 egg and 1 tablespoon of the flour to the creamed mixture. Process briefly to mix, then add the remaining eggs one at a time, each with another 1 tablespoon flour.

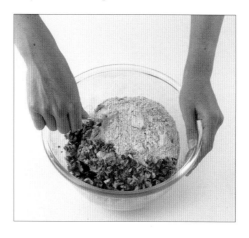

4 Scrape the mixture into a bowl and fold in the remaining flour, with the walnut pieces.

5 Grate the rind from 3 lemons and thinly pare the rind from the fourth (for decoration). Squeeze the juice from 2 lemons. Stir the grated lemon rind and juice into the mixture.

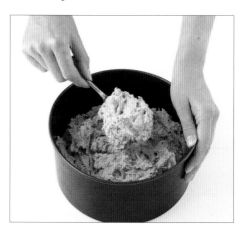

6 Spoon the batter into the prepared pan and level the top. Bake for 50–60 minutes, or until a fine skewer inserted into the center comes out clean. Cool on a wire rack. Decorate with the pared lemon rind.

NUTRITION NOTES

Per cake:	
Calories	2,845
Fat, total	163g
saturated fat	34g
polyunsaturated fat	62g
monounsaturated fat	55g
Carbohydrate	280g
sugar, total	90g
starch	190g
Fiber – NSP	34g
Sodium	1,660mg

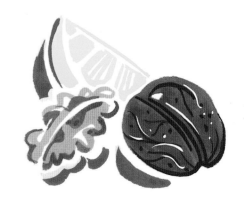

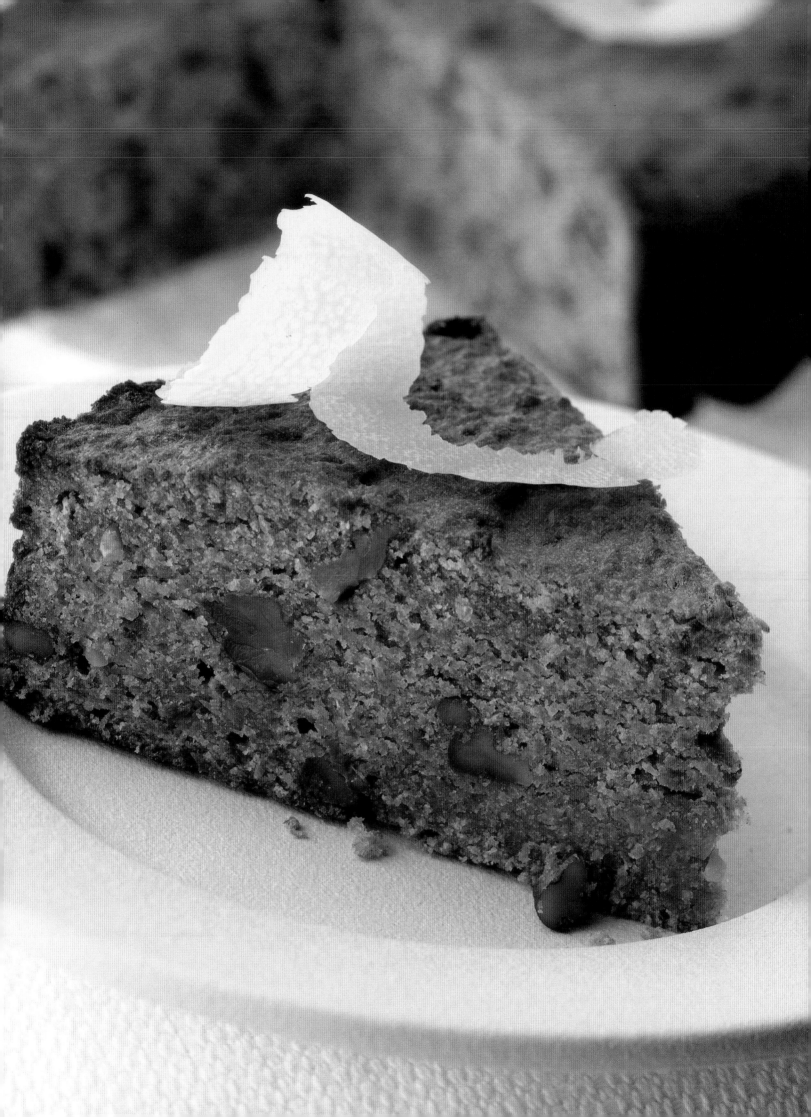

Apple Spice Cake

Moist and spicy, this is perfect for packed lunches or with coffee.

INGREDIENTS

Makes an 8-inch square cake

8 tablespoons (½ cup) low-fat spread,
   plus extra for greasing
1¼ cups pitted dates
1–2 tart eating apples or 1 cooking
   apple, about 8 ounces total
2½ teaspoons apple pie spice
½ teaspoon salt
½ cup raisins
2 eggs, beaten
1¼ cups whole-wheat flour, sifted
generous 1 cup gram flour or besan,
   sifted with 2 teaspoons baking
   powder
¾ cup unsweetened coconut milk

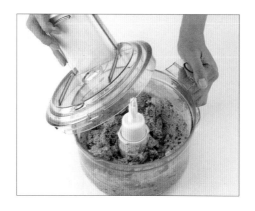

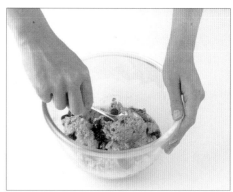

1 Preheat the oven to 350°F. Lightly grease a deep 8-inch square baking pan and line the bottom with baking parchment or waxed paper. Combine the low-fat spread and the dates in a food processor. Peel, core and grate the apple or apples and add to the low-fat spread and date mixture with the apple pie spice and salt. Process until thoroughly blended.

2 Scrape the apple and date mixture into a bowl and fold in the raisins and beaten eggs alternately with the flours, baking powder and coconut milk. Transfer to the prepared pan and smooth the surface.

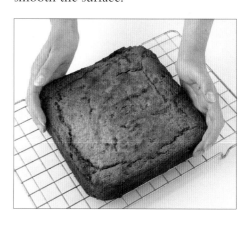

3 Bake for 30–40 minutes, until dark golden and firm. A skewer inserted into the center should come out clean. Cool the cake in the pan for 15 minutes. Turn out onto a wire rack, remove the paper and cool completely.

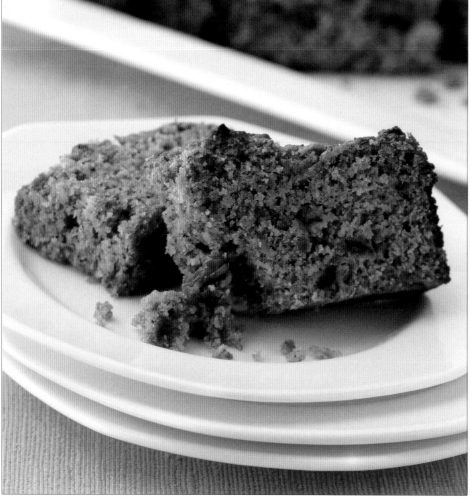

— NUTRITION NOTES —	
Per cake:	
Calories	2,036
Fat, total	72g
saturated fat	4.5g
polyunsaturated fat	18.5g
monounsaturated fat	28g
Carbohydrate	300g
sugar, total	150g
starch	147g
Fiber – NSP	34.4g
Sodium	2,412mg

Banana Bread

The very ripe bananas that are often sold cheaply at the supermarket are perfect for this tried and trusted favorite.

INGREDIENTS

Makes 1 loaf

8 tablespoons (½ cup) low-fat spread, plus extra for greasing
1 teaspoon baking soda
2 cups whole-wheat flour
2 eggs, beaten
3 very ripe bananas
2–3 tablespoons unsweetened coconut milk or soy milk

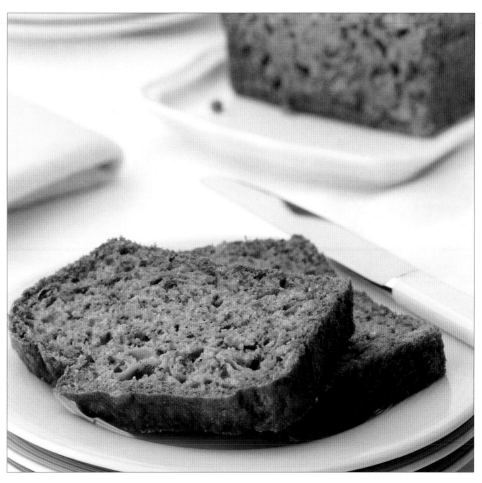

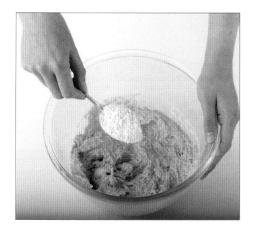

1 Preheat the oven to 350°F. Grease and line a 9 x 5-inch loaf pan. Cream the low-fat spread in a bowl until it is fluffy. Sift the baking soda with the flour, then add the dry ingredients to the creamed low-fat spread, alternately with the eggs.

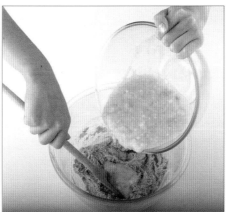

2 Peel the bananas and place them in a bowl. Mash them well, then stir them into the cake mixture. Mix in the coconut milk or soy milk.

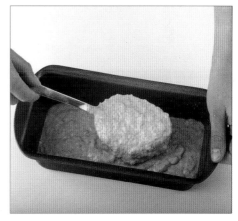

3 Spoon the batter into the prepared loaf pan and level the surface with a spoon. Bake for about 1¼ hours, or until a fine skewer inserted into the center comes out clean. Cool on a wire rack. Transfer to a serving plate, remove the paper and serve in slices.

NUTRITION NOTES

Per loaf:

Calories	1,616
Fat, total	66g
saturated fat	17.5g
polyunsaturated fat	15.2g
monounsaturated fat	26.5g
Carbohydrate	215g
sugar, total	70g
starch	145g
Fiber – NSP	23.5g
Sodium	2,320mg

VARIATION

Sunflower seeds make a good addition to banana bread. Add about ½ cup to the mixture just before baking.

Rich Fruit Cake

This makes a good Christmas or birthday cake, but its relatively high fat and natural sugar content means that it should be only an occasional treat for diabetics.

INGREDIENTS

Makes an 8-inch cake

1 large orange, quartered and seeded, but not peeled
1 large lemon, quartered and seeded, but not peeled
1 large cooking apple, cored and quartered, but not peeled
generous ½ cup pitted dates
6 tablespoons low-fat spread
6 tablespoons hazelnut butter
generous ½ cup raisins
generous ½ cup currants
generous ½ cup golden raisins
generous ½ cup pitted prunes, chopped
²⁄₃ cup broken cashews
1 teaspoon ground cinnamon
1 teaspoon grated nutmeg
½ teaspoon ground mace
½ teaspoon ground cloves
1 cup whole-wheat flour
1½ teaspoons baking powder
1 cup rolled oats, processed until smooth
3 large eggs, beaten
3–4 tablespoons unsweetened coconut milk or rice milk, if needed

---

NUTRITION NOTES	
Per cake:	
Calories	3,087
Fat, total	125g
saturated fat	30g
polyunsaturated fat	27g
monounsaturated fat	56g
Carbohydrate	440g
sugar, total	285g
starch	160g
Fiber – NSP	38g
Sodium	2,200mg

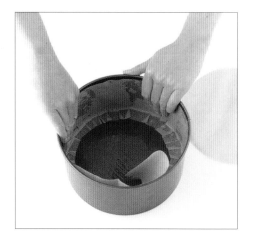

1 Preheat the oven to 300°F. Grease and line a deep 8-inch round cake pan with baking parchment.

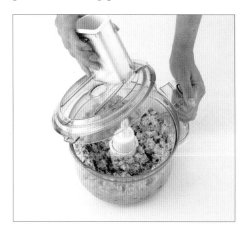

2 Combine the orange, lemon and apple in a food processor. Add the dates, low-fat spread and nut butter and process to a rough purée.

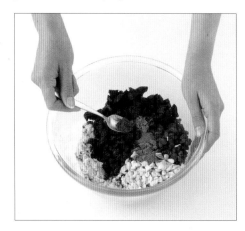

3 Scrape the mixture into a bowl and stir in the raisins, currants, golden raisins, prunes, nuts and spices.

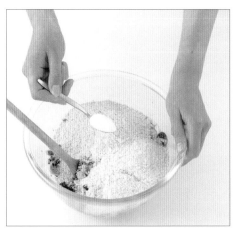

4 Stir in the flour, baking powder and rolled oats, alternately with the beaten eggs.

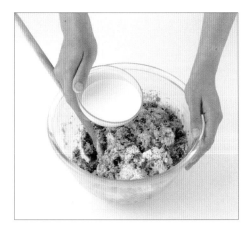

5 If the mixture seems very dry, stir in the coconut milk or rice milk.

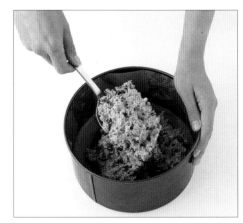

6 Spoon the cake batter into the prepared pan, level the top and bake for 1 hour, or until a fine skewer inserted into the center comes out clean. Let cool on a wire rack.

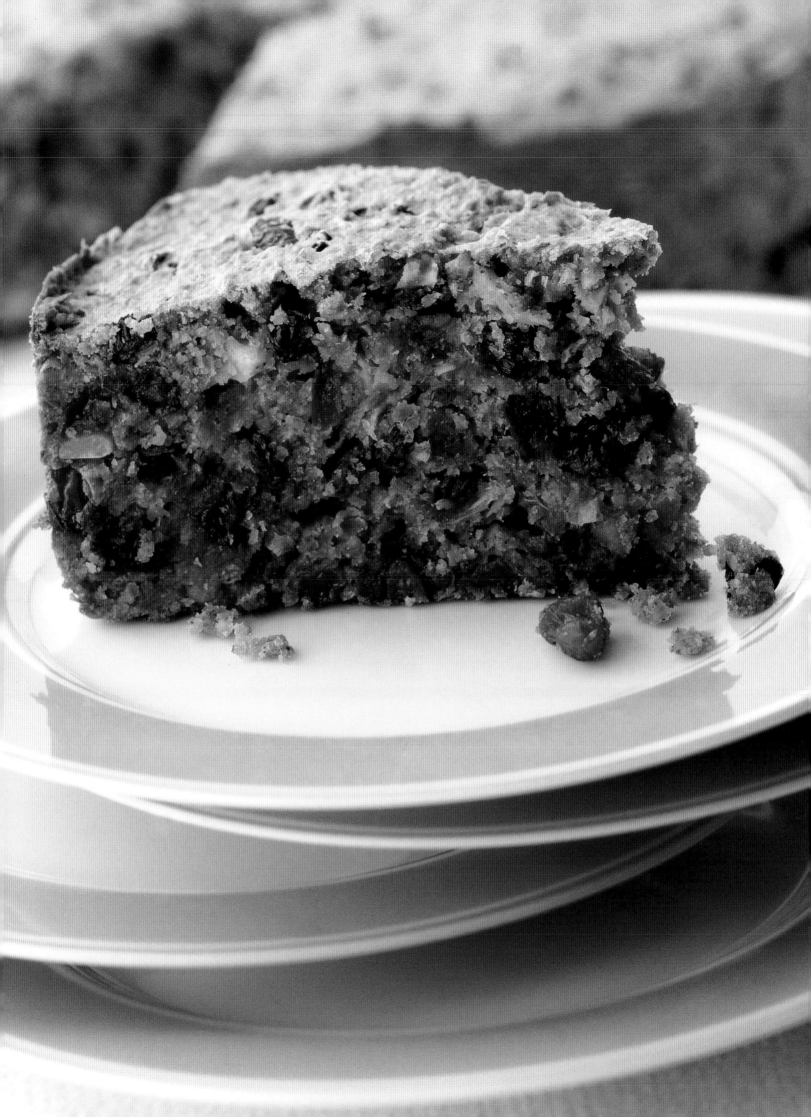

Fruit Malt Bread

INGREDIENTS

Makes 1 loaf
2¼ cups whole-wheat flour
pinch of salt
2¼ teaspoons baking powder
½ teaspoon baking soda
1 cup mixed dried fruit
1 tablespoon malt extract
1 cup skim milk
low-fat spread, to serve (optional)

COOK'S TIP

Use any combination of dried fruit you like for this bread: Choose from raisins, golden raisins and currants, or include chopped dried pears, apricots, peaches or mangoes.

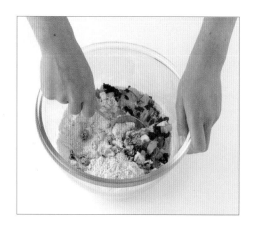

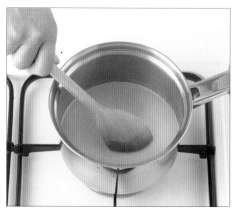

1 Preheat the oven to 325°F. Grease a 9 x 5-inch loaf pan. Line the bottom with baking parchment. Sift the flour, salt, baking powder and baking soda into a bowl. Stir in the dried fruit.

2 Heat the malt extract and milk in a small saucepan, stirring until the malt extract has dissolved. Pour into the dry ingredients and mix well.

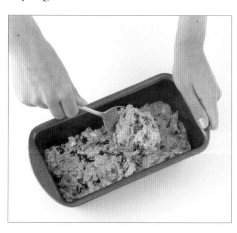

3 Spoon the mixture into the prepared pan and level the top. Bake for 45 minutes, or until a fine skewer inserted into the center comes out clean. Cool on a wire rack. Serve in slices, alone or with a low-fat spread.

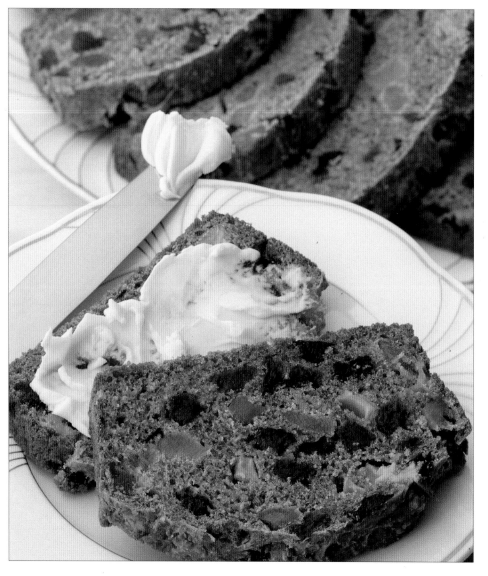

NUTRITION NOTES

Per loaf:	
Calories	1,330
Fat, total	6.5g
saturated fat	1g
polyunsaturated fat	2.5g
monounsaturated fat	7.5g
Carbohydrate	295g
sugar, total	138g
starch	155g
Fiber – NSP	26g
Sodium	1,015mg

Chocolate and Prune Cake

Thanks to the gram flour, this cake is high in soluble fiber. It is also quite high in natural sugars, though, so enjoy it only as a sometime treat.

INGREDIENTS

Makes an 8-inch cake

11 ounces bittersweet chocolate
10 tablespoons (²⁄₃ cup) low-fat spread
generous 1 cup pitted prunes, quartered
3 eggs, beaten
1¼ cups gram flour or besan, sifted
   with 2 teaspoons baking powder
½ cup unsweetened coconut milk, rice
   milk or soy milk

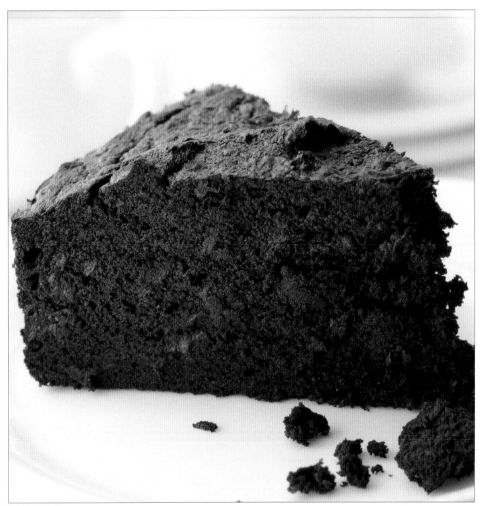

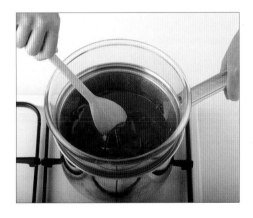

1 Preheat the oven to 350°F. Grease and line a deep 8-inch round cake pan. Melt the chocolate in a heatproof bowl over a pan of simmering water.

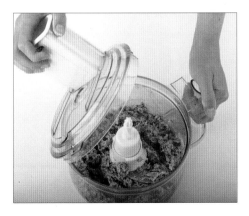

2 Mix the low-fat spread and prunes in a food processor. Process until light and fluffy, then scrape into a bowl.

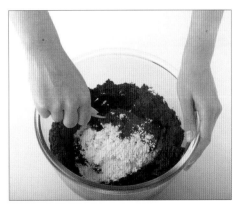

3 Gradually fold in the melted chocolate and eggs, alternately with the flour mixture. Beat in the coconut milk, rice milk or soy milk.

COOK'S TIP

Use chocolate with a high proportion of cocoa solids (70 percent) for this cake.

4 Spoon the batter into the prepared cake pan, level the surface with a spoon, then bake for 20–30 minutes, or until the cake is firm to the touch. A fine skewer inserted into the center should come out clean. Allow to cool on a wire rack before serving.

--- NUTRITION NOTES ---

Per cake:

Calories	3,178
Fat, total	174g
saturated fat	74g
polyunsaturated fat	24g
monounsaturated fat	63g
Carbohydrate	340g
sugar, total	260g
starch	72g
Fiber – NSP	35g
Sodium	2,640mg

Chocolate Brownies

Dark and full of flavor, these brownies are irresistible. They make a good afternoon treat—perfect for accompanying a cup of coffee shared with friends.

INGREDIENTS

Makes 20

10 tablespoons (²/₃ cup) low-fat spread
scant 1 cup (5 ounces) pitted dates, softened in boiling water, then drained and finely chopped
1¼ cups whole-wheat flour
3¼ teaspoons baking powder
4 tablespoons cocoa powder dissolved in 2 tablespoons hot water
4 tablespoons apple and pear spread
6 tablespoons unsweetened coconut milk
½ cup walnuts or pecans, roughly broken

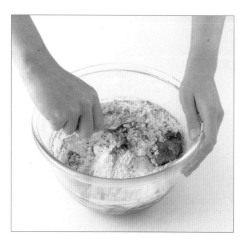

1 Preheat the oven to 325°F. Grease an 11 x 7-inch shallow baking pan. Cream the low-fat spread with the dates. Sift the flour with the baking powder, then fold into the creamed mixture, alternately with the cocoa mixture, apple and pear spread and coconut milk. Stir in the nuts.

2 Spoon the batter into the prepared pan, smooth the surface and bake for about 45 minutes, or until a fine skewer inserted into the center comes out clean. Cool for a few minutes in the pan, then cut into bars or squares. Cool on a wire rack.

NUTRITION NOTES	
Per brownie:	
Calories	91
Fat, total	5.6g
saturated fat	1.4g
polyunsaturated fat	2g
monounsaturated fat	2g
Carbohydrate	8.3g
sugar, total	3.12g
starch	5.15g
Fiber – NSP	1.3g
Sodium	142mg

Spicy Golden Raisin Muffins

Sunday breakfasts will never be the same again, once you have tried these delicious muffins! They are easy to prepare and take only a short time to bake.

INGREDIENTS

Makes 6

6 tablespoons low-fat spread
1 small egg
½ cup unsweetened coconut milk
1¼ cups whole-wheat flour
1½ teaspoons baking powder
1 teaspoon ground cinnamon
generous pinch of salt
²/₃ cup golden raisins

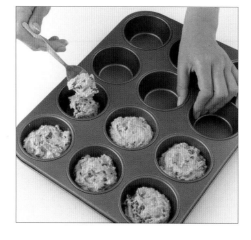

1 Preheat the oven to 375°F. Grease a muffin pan. Beat the low-fat spread, egg and coconut milk in a bowl.

2 Sift the flour, baking powder, cinnamon and salt over the mixture. Fold in, then beat well. Fold in the raisins. Spoon batter into prepared pan.

3 Bake for 20 minutes, or until the muffins have risen well and are firm to the touch. Cool slightly on a wire rack before serving.

COOK'S TIP
These muffins taste equally good at room temperature. They also freeze well, packed in freezer bags. To serve, allow them to thaw overnight, or defrost in a microwave, then warm them briefly in the oven.

NUTRITION NOTES	
Per muffin:	
Calories	123
Fat, total	6.3g
saturated fat	1.75g
polyunsaturated fat	1.35g
monounsaturated fat	2.65g
Carbohydrate	14.85g
sugar, total	14.35g
starch	0.5g
Fiber – NSP	0.4g
Sodium	278.5mg

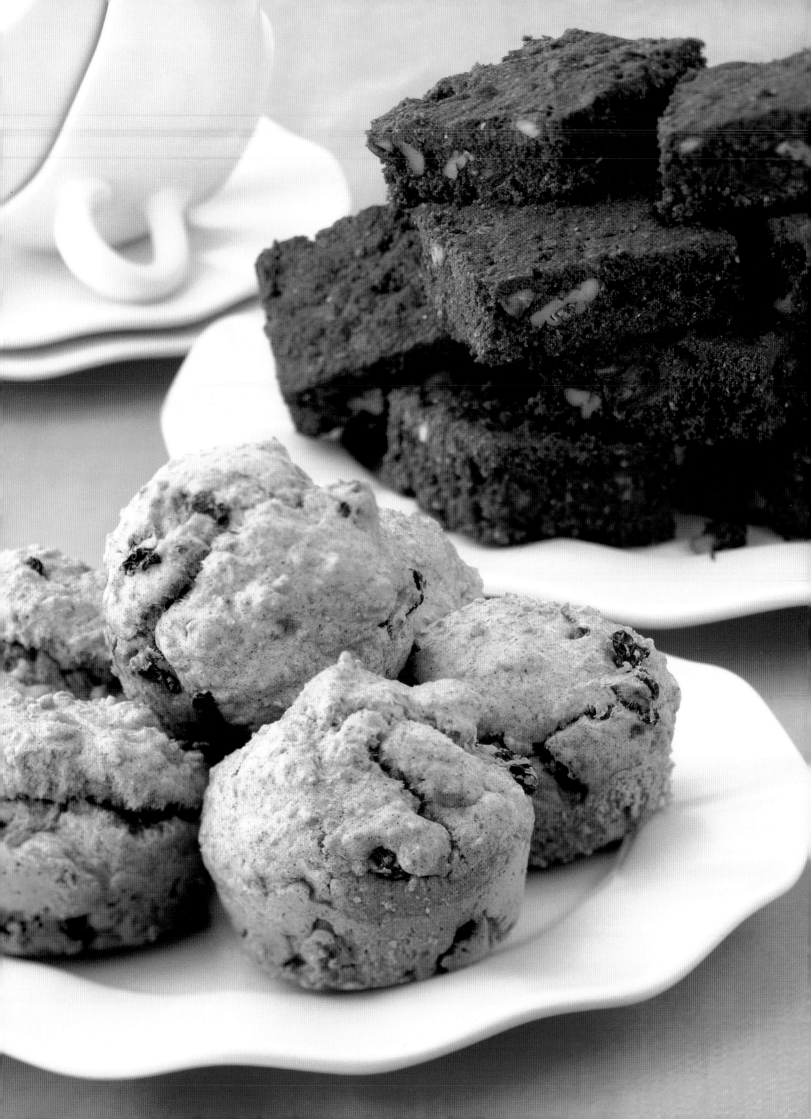

Pine Nut Cookies

Perfect for picnics and packed lunches, these cookies are really crisp and crunchy.

INGREDIENTS

Makes 16
8 tablespoons (½ cup) low-fat spread
4 tablespoons rice syrup
½ cup whole-wheat flour
2 cups rolled oats
⅔ cup (2 ounces) pine nuts

1 Preheat the oven to 350°F. Line an 8-inch shallow square baking pan with oiled foil. Melt the low-fat spread and rice syrup in a small saucepan over low heat. Off heat, stir in the flour, oats and pine nuts until well mixed.

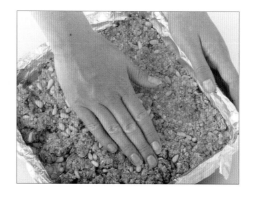

2 Scrape the mixture into the prepared pan and pat it out evenly with your fingers. Press the mixture down lightly. Bake for 25–30 minutes, until the cookies are lightly browned and crisp. Mark into squares while still warm. Cool slightly, then lift them out of the pan and cool on a wire rack.

COOK'S TIP

Do not let the syrup mixture boil or the cookies will be tacky rather than crisp.

NUTRITION NOTES

Per cookie:	
Calories	122
Fat, total	6.4g
saturated fat	1.2g
polyunsaturated fat	2.55g
monounsaturated fat	2.35g
Carbohydrate	14.3g
sugar, total	1.45g
starch	11.05g
Fiber – NSP	1.35g
Sodium	54.1mg

Ginger Cookies

INGREDIENTS

Makes 8 gingerbread men or 10–12 cookies
1 cup all-purpose flour, sifted
1½ teaspoons ground ginger
grated rind of 1 orange and 1 lemon
5 tablespoons pear and apple spread
2 tablespoons low-fat spread
16 currants and 8 raisins, to decorate (optional)

NUTRITION NOTES

Per gingerbread man:	
Calories	85
Fat, total	1.5g
saturated fat	0.4g
polyunsaturated fat	0.5g
monounsaturated fat	0.55g
Carbohydrate	17.25g
sugar, total	5.85g
starch	11.4g
Fiber – NSP	0.5g
Sodium	23.1mg

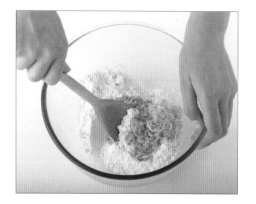

1 Mix the sifted flour, ginger and grated orange and lemon rind in a bowl. Melt the pear and apple spread and the low-fat spread in a small saucepan over low heat.

2 As soon as the pear and apple spread and low-fat spread mixture has melted, stir it into the dry ingredients. Mix to a firm dough in the bowl, then remove the dough, wrap it in plastic wrap and chill for 2–3 hours.

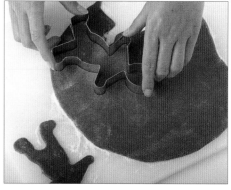

3 Preheat the oven to 350°F. Roll out the dough on a lightly floured surface to a ¼-inch thickness. Cut out men, using a cutter or template. Alternatively, stamp the dough into 10–12 rounds with a 2¾-inch cutter.

4 If making gingerbread men, give them currant eyes and raisin noses. Using the point of a knife, draw a mouth on each. Place the cookies on a lightly floured baking sheet and bake for 8–10 minutes. Cool on a wire rack.

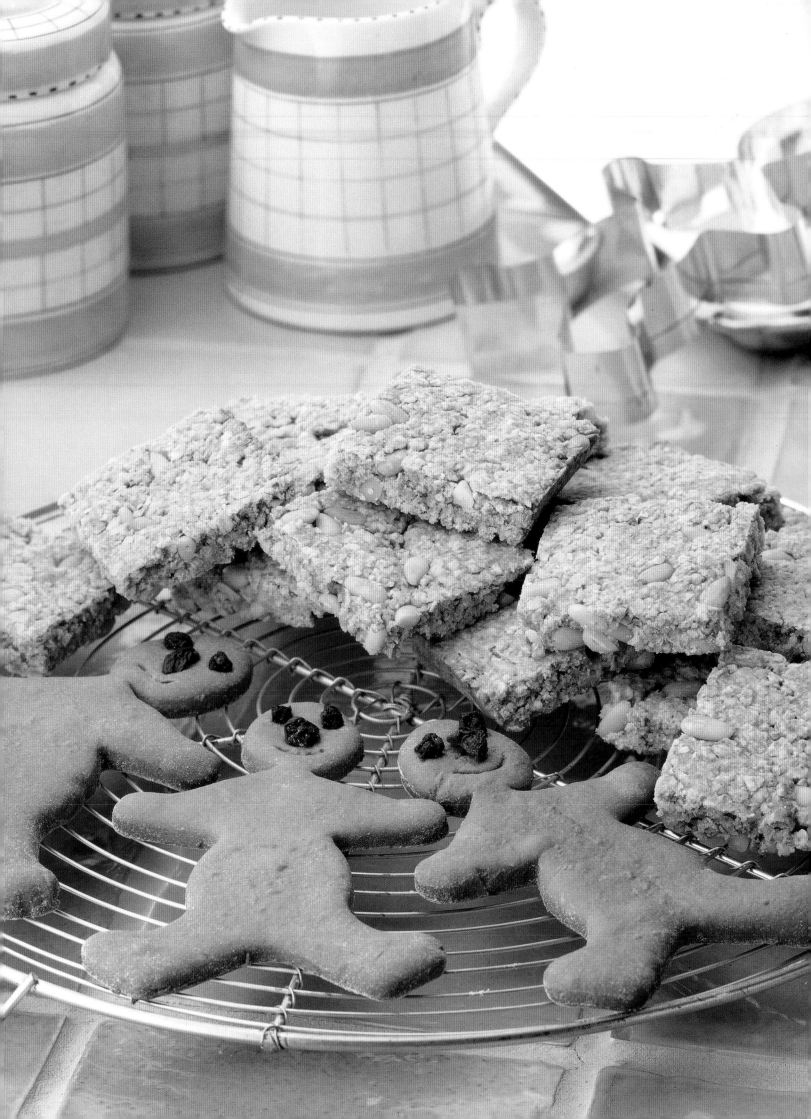

Fruit and Nut Chocolates

When beautifully boxed, these make perfect presents.

INGREDIENTS

Makes 20

$\frac{1}{3}$ cup (2 ounces) pitted prunes or
  dried apricots
$\frac{1}{3}$ cup golden raisins or raisins
2 tablespoons dried apples, figs or dates
$\frac{1}{3}$ cup sliced almonds
$\frac{1}{4}$ cup hazelnuts or walnuts
2–4 tablespoons lemon juice
2 ounces bittersweet chocolate

1 Chop the fruit and nuts in a food processor or blender until fairly small. Add 2 tablespoons lemon juice and process again to mix. Scrape the mixture into a bowl, taste and add more lemon juice if needed.

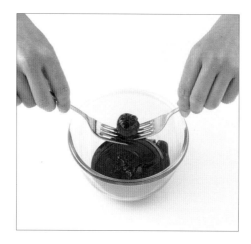

2 Melt the chocolate in a heatproof bowl over a pan of simmering water. Roll the fruit mixture into small balls. Using two forks or tongs, roll each ball in the melted chocolate, then place on oiled foil to cool and set. If the chocolate becomes too solid to work with, reheat it gently.

NUTRITION NOTES	
Per chocolate:	
Calories	42
Fat, total	2.3g
saturated fat	0.55g
polyunsaturated fat	0.8g
monounsaturated fat	0.8g
Carbohydrate	4.95g
sugar, total	4.85g
starch	0.05g
Fiber – NSP	0.5g
Sodium	1.9mg

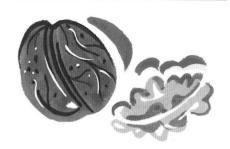

Apple and Date Balls

INGREDIENTS

Makes 20

$2\frac{1}{4}$ pounds cooking apples or pears
$\frac{2}{3}$ cup (4 ounces) pitted dates
1 cup apple juice
1 teaspoon ground cinnamon
$\frac{1}{2}$ cup finely chopped walnuts

NUTRITION NOTES	
Per ball:	
Calories	47
Fat, total	1.8g
saturated fat	0.15g
polyunsaturated fat	1.25g
monounsaturated fat	0.3g
Carbohydrate	7.6g
sugar, total	7.6g
starch	0g
Fiber – NSP	1g
Sodium	1.9mg

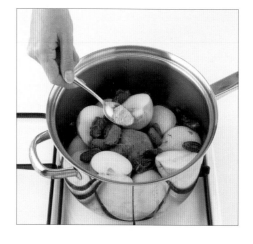

1 Halve and core the unpeeled fruit and place in a large, heavy saucepan. Add the dates, apple juice and ground cinnamon. Cook over very low heat, stirring occasionally, for 4–6 hours, or until the mixture forms a dry paste. Scrape into a bowl and cool, then roll the mixture into bite-size balls. Toast the nuts under the broiler until golden.

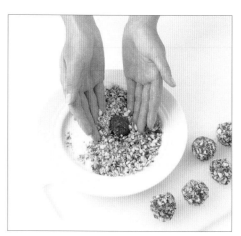

2 Coat the balls in the nuts. Twist each ball in a candy wrapper or cellophane; store in an airtight box.

VARIATION
Use half ground cinnamon and half ground ginger instead of the 1 teaspoon cinnamon.

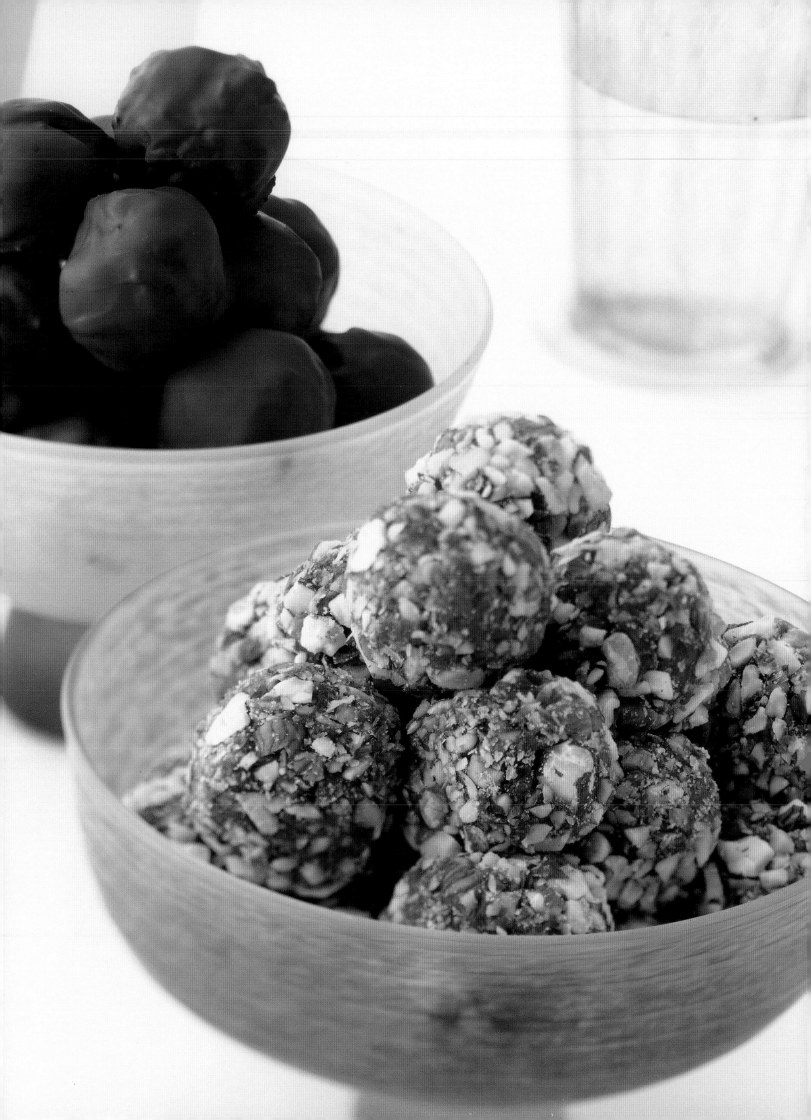

Whole-Wheat Cheese Biscuits

These are very good warm for breakfast or as a snack.

INGREDIENTS

Makes 15

4 cups (1 pound) whole-wheat flour
pinch of salt
2 teaspoons baking powder
4 ounces Parmesan cheese, finely grated
4 tablespoons (¼ cup) sunflower
   margarine
⅔–1¼ cups buttermilk (see
   Cook's Tip)

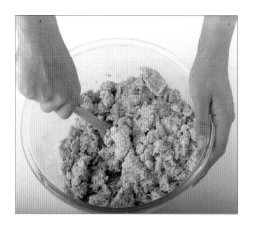

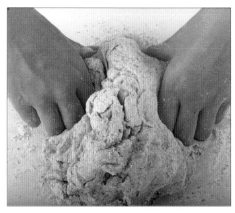

1 Preheat the oven to 400°F. Mix the flour, salt, baking powder and Parmesan cheese in a bowl and rub in the margarine with your fingertips until the mixture resembles bread crumbs. Working quickly and lightly, stir in enough of the buttermilk to make a moist dough.

2 Pat out the dough on a lightly floured board to a thickness of about 1½ inches.

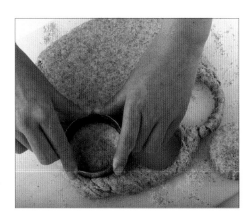

3 Using a 2¾-inch cutter, cut out 15 rounds. Place the rounds on a floured baking sheet and bake for about 10 minutes. The exact cooking time will depend on the height of the biscuits. They should be well risen and lightly browned. Serve warm, cut in half, with a little sunflower margarine.

— COOK'S TIP —

If you don't have buttermilk on hand, sour skim milk by stirring in a generous squeeze of lemon juice. Let the mixture stand for about 10 minutes before using it.

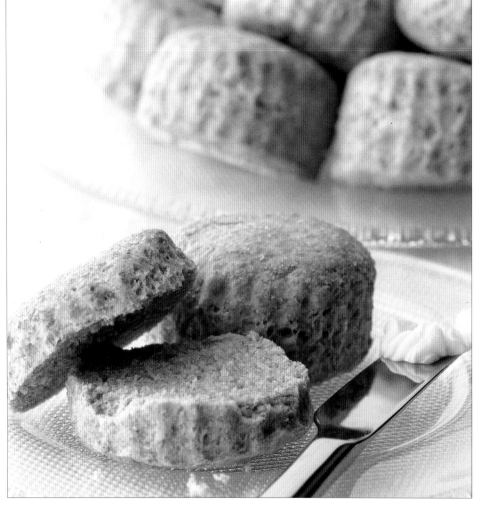

NUTRITION NOTES	
Per biscuit:	
Calories	160
Fat, total	5.95g
saturated fat	2.25g
polyunsaturated fat	1.55g
monounsaturated fat	1.7g
Carbohydrate	20.4g
sugar, total	1.65g
starch	18.8g
Fiber – NSP	2.7g
Sodium	196.6mg

Information File

FURTHER READING

The Art of Cooking for the Diabetic by Mary Abbott Hess, L.H.D., M.S., R.D., F.A.D.A.—Contemporary Books

How to Cook for People with Diabetes American Diabetes Association—American Diabetes Association

The Diabetic's Healthy Exchanges Cookbook by Jo Anna M. Lund—Healthy Exchanges Inc.

Diabetic Meals in 30 Minutes—or Less! by Robyn Webb—American Diabetes Association

Diabetic Low-Fat ad No-Fat Meals in Minutes by M.J. Smith, R.D.—Chronimed Publishing

HELPFUL ORGANIZATIONS

The American Diabetes Association
1660 Duke Street
Alexandria, VA 22314
(800) 232 3472

Juvenile Diabetes Foundation
432 Park Avenue
New York, NY 10016
(800) 533 8590

American Association of Diabetes Educators
Suite 1240
444 N. Michigan Avenue
Chicago, IL 60606 6995
(800) 877 1600
Pretaped nutrition messages and referrals to a local registered dietician for individual counseling.

International Diabetes Center
3800 Park Nicollet Blvd.
Minneapolis, MN 55416
(612) 993 3393
Publishes books on diabetes; offers educational programs; information on upcoming conferences and additional information on diabetes.

SHORT GLOSSARY OF BASIC TERMS

Adrenaline—hormone produced by the adrenal gland to combat physical or nervous stress.

Arteriosclerosis—hardening or clogging of the arteries.

Blood glucose—glucose level in the blood (also known as blood sugar), usually elevated in the case of diabetics.

Cystitis—inflammation of the bladder.

Diabetes Mellitus—condition where the blood sugar level is above normal.

Diuretics—pills that increase the flow of urine.

Glucose—simple sugar found in carbohydrates providing one of the main energy sources for the body.

Glycogen—the form in which glucose is stored in the blood.

Glycosuria—sugar or glucose in the urine.

Hyperglycemia—too much sugar or glucose in the blood.

Hypoglycemia—too little sugar or glucose in the blood.

Insulin—hormone produced in the pancreas, which allows glucose to enter the bloodstream.

Insulin Dependent Diabetes or Type I—a condition in which the pancreas stops producing insulin. The only treatment is injected insulin.

Insulin receptor—site on the surface of a cell into which the insulin "docks" in order to allow the glucose to enter through the cell walls.

Juvenile-onset diabetes—diabetes starting in youth that is nearly always insulin dependent.

Ketoacidosis—severe excess of glucose in the blood due to a severe insulin deficiency causing fat break-down and ketone formation.

Ketones—products that result from fat breakdown that in turn results from severe insulin deficiency. They smell of acetone and are a symptom of severe hyperglycemia.

Maturity onset diabetes—diabetes that affects people over 30 and that is not usually insulin dependent.

Neuropathy—an abnormality in the functioning of the nerves. Autonomic neuropathy is partial failure of the nerves controlling automatic body functions. Peripheral neuropathy means that the nerves in the arms and legs are affected.

Non-Insulin Dependent Diabetes or Type II—a condition where the pancreas is still producing insulin, but either it is not producing enough or it is not acting very effectively. Can usually be treated through diet and glucose-lowering drugs.

Pancreas—a gland that is found behind the stomach but in front of the spine. The pancreas produces insulin and other digestive hormones.

Polydipsia—drinking large amounts of water.

Polyuria—passing excessive amounts of urne on a frequent basis.

Retinopathy—abnormality of the retina, often caused by diabetes.

Index